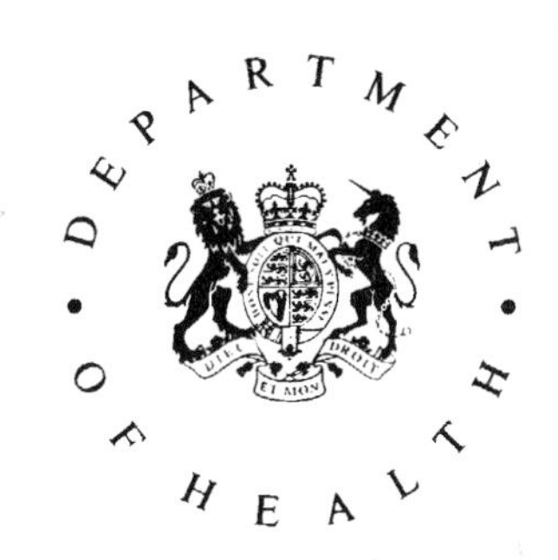

Health Related Behaviour

An Epidemiological Overview

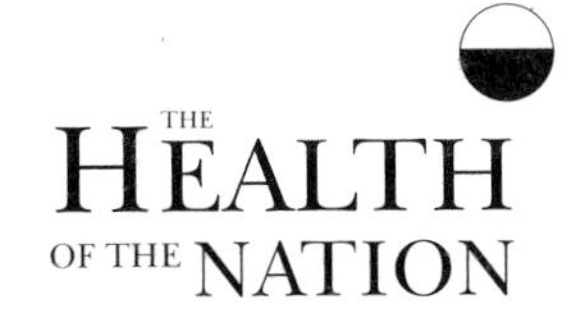

CENTRAL HEALTH MONITORING UNIT EPIDEMIOLOGICAL OVERVIEW SERIES London: THE STATIONERY OFFICE
Commissioned by Central Health Monitoring Unit from Office of Population Censuses and Surveys

Second Impression

ISBN 0 11 321976 8

FOREWORD

The Health of the Nation White Paper published in 1992 emphasised the fact that an individual's health is dependent, at least in part, on their own chosen lifestyle. This underlines the key role of *behaviour* and I believe that an understanding of health related behaviours and the factors which influence them (ie "behavioural epidemiology") is one of the most important public health issues for the future. It is for this reason that the Department of Health (DH) has itself embarked on an initiative in this area which will be taken forward in collaboration between its Health Promotion and Research and Development Divisions.

An essential preliminary to this process is reviewing existing knowledge. For this reason the Department of Health's Central Health Monitoring Unit (CHMU) has commissioned the present overview through the Office of Population Censuses and Surveys. It is the latest in a series produced by CHMU and it describes how behaviours related to the 5 Health of the Nation key areas are distributed across time, place and person. This, and other such reviews which have also been commissioned, will pinpoint specific sub-groups who need to be targeted for health promotion interventions (eg the young), identify gaps in information, and generate hypotheses which can then be tested through further work.

The overview is complementary to a number of other projects including the Health Education Authority's Health Education Monitoring Survey[1], and DH's Health Survey for England[2]. I believe that this overview, and the others mentioned above, represent a major contribution to public health policy and will, therefore, be of interest to all those centrally and at a local level who are concerned with health promotion and the prevention of disease.

Sir Kenneth Calman
Chief Medical Officer

[1]Bridgwood A, Malbon G, Lader D, Matheson J. Health in England 1995: What people know, what people think, what people do. London: HMSO, 1996.
[2]Colhoun H, Prescott Clarke P (eds.) Wei Dong, Hedges B, Lampe F, Taylor A (principal contributors). Health Survey for England 1994. London: HMSO, 1996.

ACKNOWLEDGEMENTS

This overview was commissioned by the Department of Health (DH) through Jil Matheson and Karen Dunnell of the Office of Population Censuses and Surveys (OPCS). The overview was produced by external consultants, Alison Walker and Elizabeth Hoinville under the supervision of Sunjai Gupta of DH's Central Health Monitoring Unit (CHMU). It was carried out in consultation with other parts of DH (including other members of CHMU, Androulla Michael of Health Promotion Division, Liza Catan of Research and Development Division, and members of Statistics Division and the relevant Policy Divisions). The work has been carried out with the assistance of organisations outside DH including OPCS, the Health Education Authority (HEA), the Ministry of Agriculture, Fisheries and Food (MAFF), the Department of Trade and Industry (DTI), and also selected individual experts including Michael Farrell at the Maudsley Hospital.

CONTENTS

SUMMARY

This overview brings together in one publication up-to-date information on health related behaviour. It concentrates on behaviours relevant to the five Health of the Nation key areas, presenting data for England as a whole. An appendix gives some summary figures for regions.

Diet

* The percentage of food energy obtained from total fat and saturated fatty acids showed almost no variation with any of the socio-demographic factors presented
* Dietary behaviour varied with most socio-demographic factors. For example
* 34% of people aged 75 or more reported using butter or hard margarine, compared with 18% of 16–24 year olds
* 44% of women in social classes IV & V reported using whole milk, compared with 27% in social classes I & II

Alcohol Consumption

* 26% of men and 12% of women in England drank more than the recommended sensible level of alcohol
* 39% of divorced and separated men drank over the sensible level compared with 24% of married men
* 1 in 7 road accident fatalities occurred in accidents where the driver had illegal blood alcohol levels

Physical activity

* More men than women were regularly physically active
* 1 in 4 young women and 1 in 6 young men took no regular physical activity
* Among unemployed men, 34% took no regular physical activity compared with 22% of men in work
* Similar proportions of men and women were sedentary

Smoking

* 29% of men and 27% of women were smokers
* From the age of 14, girls were more likely to smoke than boys and there was no evidence of a decline in girls smoking
* Prevalence of smoking was higher among people in the manual social classes, the unemployed, people who were widowed, separated or divorced, and Bangladeshi men

* Smoking during pregnancy was five times more common among women in social class V than among women in social class I

Screening for cancer

* 72% of women aged 50–64 who were invited to breast screening were screened
* 64% of women aged 20–64 who were invited to cervical screening were screened; the highest response was among women aged 35–39
* Low attendance for cervical screening was reported by Asian women, particularly Pakistani and Bangladeshi women

Sunburn

* 16% of men and 14% of women reported at least one episode of sunburn in the past year that had lasted more than a day

Suicide

* Suicide was three times more common among men than among women
* The suicide rate was rising among young men
* Suicide rates were higher in the elderly than the young but rates for older people were falling
* The suicide rate was particularly high among young Asian women compared with young women overall

Sexual behaviour

* Experience of first sexual intercourse was occurring at a younger age; the median age for women aged under 25 was 17 compared with 21 for women aged 55–59
* 14% of men and 7% of women reported 2 or more heterosexual partners in the previous year
* First sexual intercourse occurred at a younger age among people in the manual social classes
* There was no social class trend with number of partners
* 37% of men and 26% of women with a heterosexual partner reported using condoms
* Condom use was higher among young people, men in social class V, and single men and women

Drug misuse

* Sharing of injecting equipment among drug misusers has declined since 1987

Accidents

* 41% of deaths among 15–24 year old men were due to accidents
* Three quarters of accidental deaths among 15–24 year olds were due to road accidents

* Among children under 15, road accidents accounted for about half of accidental deaths
* The casualty rate in road accidents has declined
* Deaths in accidents at home accounted for 40% of all accidental deaths and death rates were higher among boys than girls and higher among men than women except for those aged 75 or more
* Falls were the most frequent cause of accidental death among people aged 65 or more
* Death rates in fires were highest among people aged 60 or more and were high among people born in the Indian sub-continent, the Caribbean and African Commonwealth countries
* Fatalities in fires decreased from 15 to 11 per million population between 1983 and 1993 but non-fatal casualties increased slightly
* 35% of deaths in fires occurred in fires started by smokers' materials
* 50% of homes in Great Britain had a smoke alarm

LIST OF FIGURES

LIST OF TABLES

INTRODUCTION

The purpose of this overview is to provide a reference document which brings together a broad range of up-to-date statistics on health-related behaviour. Where appropriate, these statistics have been presented in the form of "user friendly" graphics, and key sources of data and further information have been identified wherever possible. The overview is the latest in a series of such documents that have been produced or commissioned by the Department of Health's Central Health Monitoring Unit. Earlier items in the series have included overviews on the health of the elderly, coronary heart disease, stroke and asthma.

The document should be seen in the context of the "Health of the Nation" White Paper which emphasised the importance of lifestyle and behaviour as determinants of health. The overview is part of an initiative on "behavioural epidemiology" (ie the study of health-related *behaviour* and the factors which influence them) which has been initiated by the Department of Health. It concentrates on behaviour (relevant to the five Health of the Nation key areas), but has been carried out in consultation with the Health Education Authority (HEA) which will be focusing on knowledge, attitudes and beliefs related to such behaviour.

Where appropriate the overview has concentrated on data for England but where such data were not readily available or where it was felt the comparisons were appropriate, data for the other UK countries have been included.

The overview has been commissioned by the Department of Health (DH) through the Office of Population Censuses and Surveys (OPCS), and its target audience includes members of the relevant DH policy branches, as well as DH expert committees. However, the overview is also aimed at experts and interested groups outside DH including organisations specifically concerned with health, clinicians, nurses, researchers, public health doctors and those working in the fields of disease prevention and health promotion.

It is, of course, difficult to produce a single document which fully caters for the needs of such a wide ranging audience, and the composition of the overview inevitably, therefore, represents something of a compromise. For example, although many of those at whom it is aimed are already familiar with the technical terms employed in the overview, a glossary of selected items has been provided in case clarification is required. Similarly a minimum amount of text has been provided to assist with interpretation of the graphics. However, the level of detail provided may fall short of that which some readers may prefer, and the text is deliberately restricted to objective descriptions of the data rather than an attempt at inference or analysis of causal relationships. Nor has any attempt been made to provide a review of the academic literature on the subject (which includes many local studies, unlike the overview which tends to focus on national data).

Despite these restrictions we hope that the document will provide a useful reference source and future editions may provide further up-dating of the relevant statistics as appropriate.

HEALTH RELATED BEHAVIOURS INCLUDED IN THIS OVERVIEW

The Health of the Nation (HON) White Paper (1992) set targets within each of five key areas against which to monitor improvements in the nation's health. The strategy emphasises disease prevention and health promotion as ways in which improvements in health can be secured. Investigation of the health related behaviour of individuals contributes to this strategy.

The behaviours selected for this overview reflect the aim of the targets. In some cases, such as smoking and drinking, behaviours form the targets within the Health of the Nation, but in other key areas the choice was not so clear.

In these cases the selection was based on the content of the HON White Paper and discussions with experts in the Department of Health and elsewhere. At least one behaviour was selected for each key area but some behaviours related to more than one area. These relationships are shown in Matrix 1.

The overview presents data for each of the behaviour groups in separate sections with a commentary. A section summarising the health behaviours of each socio-demographic group is also included.

SUMMARY OF THE INDICATORS USED

Diet

% of food energy from total fat

% of food energy from saturated fatty acids

type of milk used

type of fat spread used

% eating fruit daily

% eating vegetables/salad daily

% eating bread more than once a day

Alcohol Consumption

% of men drinking more than 21 units of alcohol a week and of women drinking more than 14 units a week

number of injuries/deaths in alcohol-related road traffic accidents

Physical Activity

% engaging in vigorous intensity activity at least 3x20 minutes per week

% engaging in at least moderate intensity activity at least 5x30 minutes per week

% sedentary (less than 1x30 minutes per week of at least moderate activity)

Smoking

prevalence of cigarette smoking among men and women 16+

cigarettes released for home consumption

prevalence of cigarette smoking among 11–15 year olds

% of pregnant women smokers who give up when pregnant

Screening for Cancer

uptake of invitation to breast screening among women aged 50–64

uptake of invitation to cervical screening

Excessive Exposure to Sun

prevalence of sunburn

Suicide

overall suicide rate

suicide rate among severely mentally ill

Sexual Behaviour

age at first intercourse

number of sexual partners

% using condoms in past year

number of conceptions among under 16s

Drug Misuse

% of injecting drug misusers sharing injecting equipment

Accidents

accidental death rate
casualties/fatalities in road accidents
casualties/fatalities in fires
casualties/fatalities in the home
% of households with smoke alarms

MATRIX 1

HEALTH OF THE NATIONAL KEY AREAS AND RELEVANT BEHAVIOUR

Behaviour	CHD and Stroke	Cancers	Mental Illness	HIV/AIDS Sexual Health	Accidents
% of food energy from total fat	+	+			
saturated fatty acids	+	+			
consumption of specific foods					
milk, spreads, fruit/veg, bread	+	+			
% of men drinking > 21 units and					
of women drinking > 14 units/week	+	+	+	+	+
casualties/fatalities in road					
accidents involving alcohol					
% engaging in vigorous activity					
at least 3x20 mins/week	+				
at least moderate activity			+		+
% at least 5x30 mins/week	+				
% less 1x30 mins/week	+				
prevalence of cigarette smoking					
among men and women 16+	+	+			+
prevalence of cigarette smoking					
among boys & girls 11–15+	+	+			+
% of pregnant women smokers					
who give up while pregnant	+	+			
% of women aged 50–64 taking up					
invitation to breast screening		+			
% of women taking up invitation					
to cervical screening		+			
prevalence of sunburn		+			
overall suicide rate			+		
suicide rate among severely mentally ill			+		
age at first intercourse		+		+	
no. of sexual partners		+		+	
use of condoms in past year		+		+	
no. of conceptions under age 16		+		+	
% of injecting drug misusers					
sharing injecting equipment				+	
% of accidental deaths					+
casualties/deaths in					
road accidents					+
fires					+
the home					+
% households with smoke alarm					+

This matrix does not necessarily imply causation. The nature of the relationships between the Health of the Nation key areas and behaviours varies.

AN OVERVIEW OF BEHAVIOUR WITHIN SOCIO-DEMOGRAPHIC GROUPS

This section summarises how the health related behaviours selected for this overview were represented in different groups within the population. A summary matrix can be found at the end of the section.

Younger adults With the exception of a few behaviours, people in the younger age groups tended to engage in behaviours damaging to health to a greater extent than those in the middle or older age range. Smoking was most prevalent among 20–24 year olds; drinking above the sensible level was more frequent among the young who were also more likely to die in an alcohol related traffic accident. The proportion of deaths due to accidents was highest among 15–24 year olds. Younger adults also had the highest casualty rates for road accidents and one of the highest rates for casualties in fires.

Although physical activity was generally higher among younger people this was not so for young women aged 16–24. Younger people were less likely than older people to eat fruit, vegetables or salad on a daily basis or bread more than once a day. Sunburn was more prevalent among young people. In terms of sexual behaviour, younger people had intercourse at an earlier age than older people did and they had more partners on average, but they were more likely to use a condom. The suicide rate rose among younger men.

Older people Prevalence rates of most of the major health related behaviours (smoking, alcohol consumption, sexual behaviour and diet) were generally lower among older people. The two main areas where they did not fare so well are physical activity and accidents. Older people were active less often and more likely to be sedentary than people in the younger and middle age ranges. They had the highest death rates from accidents overall and for road accidents and fires. They also had the highest casualty rates for injuries caused by fires and households headed by someone over the age of 75 were the least likely to have a smoke alarm fitted.

Within the age range 20–64 a smaller proportion of the older women than of those in the middle of the range had attended for cervical screening. Attendance for breast screening was fairly high among 50–64 year old women. Suicide was more prevalent among older women and still had a high rate for older men although the rate fell for both older men and women.

Children and young teenagers The data for smoking among teenagers do not suggest any reduction in prevalence compared with their older counterparts, and with a third of 15 year old boys reporting that they drank at least once a week it seems likely this was also the case for drinking. The conception rate among girls under 16 was 9.3 per 1,000 girls. Children and young teenagers were more at risk from accidents in the home than other age groups and over a third of the deaths in children aged 5–15 were as a result of accidents. Very young children (under 5) also had high death rates from fires.

Men Slightly more men than women smoked cigarettes. Among the under 16s a greater proportion of girls smoked than boys. More than twice as many men as women drank more than the recommended sensible level and more boys reported drinking at least once a week. Men were less likely to eat salad, vegetables or fruit on a daily basis but more of them said they ate bread more than once a day.

In terms of sexual behaviour, men tended to experience intercourse earlier than women and to have more partners. More of them reported using condoms. Sunburn was slightly more common among men than women. Death through accidents was more frequent among men and this was found both for road accidents and fires. Men were also much more likely than women to commit suicide.

Women More women than men exhibited health-conscious dietary behaviour (more frequent fruit and vegetable eating and a smaller proportion using whole milk). Women, in particular young women, participated in physical activity less regularly than men, but, from age 24 onwards, women were slightly less likely than men to be totally sedentary. Older women were more likely than older men to report having an accident in the home and older women had the highest death rate from accidents in the home.

Socio-economic groups People in the manual groups were more likely to smoke cigarettes than those in the non-manual groups, and pregnant women smokers in the manual groups were less likely to stop smoking. For the other behaviours for which social class data are available the distinction between manual and non-manual groups tended not to be so clearly defined. Drinking in excess of the sensible level was more common among women in the non-manual groups but, among men, it was those in the employers and managers group and the unskilled whose alcohol consumption was higher.

Dietary behaviour varied with social class with those in social classes IV and V eating fruit and vegetables less often and being more likely to use whole milk. There was no difference between the classes in the percentage of food energy provided by total fat or by saturates. Men in the manual groups were more likely to be regularly active or totally sedentary. Activity levels included occupational activity which contributes to this finding. Lower social class was associated with deaths from accidents especially among children under 15.

Experience of first intercourse was at a lower age among people from the manual groups but there was no clear social class pattern with respect to the number of partners or condom use, although the use of condoms was more frequently reported by people in social class V.

Unemployment Data regarding employment were not published for many of the behaviours selected for this overview (although in some cases the data have been collected and are available for further analysis). Unemployed men were more likely to smoke and less likely to be physically active than men in work. Among women those who were unemployed were more likely to smoke.

Widowed, separated and divorced people This group was more likely to smoke than married or single people. Divorced and separated men were more likely to drink over the sensible level. Widowed, separated and divorced people had more sexual partners in the past year and were less likely to use condoms than single people. Suicides were more frequent in this group.

Ethnic minority groups The prevalence of smoking was very low among Asian women but high among Bangladeshi men. Fewer of the teenagers from ethnic minority groups smoked than among the general population. Reported attendance for screening for cervical cancer was lower than average among Asian women. Suicide rates were higher than average among people born in the African Commonwealth countries and considerably higher among young Asian women. Experience of first intercourse was at a younger age among black males but at an older than average age among Asian men and women.

Regional variation Most behaviours varied to some extent with region but very few showed a general pattern by geographical area. The exceptions to this were

smoking among women – higher in the north
drinking over the sensible level among men – higher in the north
frequent consumption of fruit or vegetables – lower in the north
frequent consumption of bread – higher in the north
response to breast or cervical screening – lower in the Thames regions

Secular trends

Increasing	drinking above the sensible level (men 45+) smoking among girls (slight increase) suicide (young men) casualties in fires consumption of low fat milk response to cervical screening use of condoms (reported by women) smoke alarms fitted
Decreasing	smoking overall smoking among boys consumption of whole milk suicide (older men and women) deaths and injuries in road accidents deaths in fires accidents in the home consumption of vegetables and salad
No apparent trend	smoking among young adults drinking above the sensible level (men overall and women) physical activity
Levelling off after increase	consumption of fruit
Levelling off after decrease	consumption of bread

SUMMARY MATRIX	% of food energy from total fat & saturates	type of fat spread	type of milk used	% eating fruit daily	% eating veg/salad daily	% eating bread more than once a day	% drinking over sensible levels	casualties/ deaths in alcohol related road accidents	% engaging in regular vigorous exercise	% engaging in regular moderate exercise
Age	no marked variation	butter/hard margarine higher among older	whole milk higher among older	increases with age	generally higher among older	increases with age	decreases with age	higher among younger drivers	decreases steeply with age	decreases with age except for women aged 16–24
Sex	no marked variation	no marked variation	whole milk lower among women	higher among women	higher among women	higher among men	higher among men, regular drinking higher among boys	*	higher among men	higher among men
Secular Trend	Slight decrease in saturates	*	whole milk decreasing low fat milk increasing	levelling out after increase (average amount)	decreasing (average amount)	levelling out after decrease (average amount)	men: no change since 1986 women: slight increase	decreasing	no marked variation between 1990 and 1994	*
Socio-Economic	no marked variation	no marked variation	whole milk higher in manual cases	highest in groups I and II	highest in groups I and II	men: higher among manual group women: no variation	men: higher in emp/manager & unskilled women: higher in non-manual group	*	men: higher in manual groups women: no variation	higher in manual groups
Economic Activity	no marked variation	*	*	*	*	*	no variation	*	*	men: higher among employed women: no variation
Marital Status Household Type	% total fat slightly higher in 3+ adult households	*	*	*	*	*	lower among widowed higher among sep/divorced	*	*	*
Ethnic Group	*	*	*	*	*	*	*	*	*	*
Region	men: higher in north women: some variation	some variation	some variation	lower in north	lower in north	higher in north	men: higher in north women: some variation	*	some variation	*

SUMMARY MATRIX (cont.)	prevalence of cigarette smoking among 16+	prevalence of cigarette smoking among 11–15	% of smokers who give up when pregnant	% uptake of invitation to breast screening	uptake of invitation to cervical screening	prevalence of sunburn	overall suicide rate	% using condoms in past year	age at first intercourse	% with 2+ partners in past year. 10+ partners in lifetime
Age	highest among 20–24 then decreases	increases steeply with age	*	*	highest among 35–39	decreases with age	men: highest among 85+ and 35–44 women: higher among older	decreases with age	younger among younger people	2+ year: highest in 16–24 10+ life: highest in 25–34
Sex	slightly higher among men	higher among girls	NA	NA	NA	higher among men	higher among men	higher among men	older among women	higher among men
Secular Trend	decreasing overall but not among young	boys: decreasing girls: slight increase	increased between 85 and 90	no difference between 91/92 and 92/93	indication of increase	*	men: increasing particularly young men women: decreasing	increasing slowly (women)	*	*
Socio-Economic	higher among manual groups	no variation	higher among non-manual groups	*	*	men: no variation women: higher among I and II	men: some variation women: *	highest among class V but no man./non-man. trend	younger among manual groups	some variation
Economic Activity	higher among unemployed	NA	*	*	*	no variation	*	*	*	*
Marital Status Household Type	higher among wid/sep/div lower among married	NA	*	*	*	higher among single and married with children	highest among wid/sep/div. lowest among married	highest among single	*	higher among wid/sep/div
Ethnic Group	higher among Bangladeshi men very low among Asian women	higher among white children	*	*	reported screening lower among Asian women	*	particularly high among young Asian women	*	older for Asian men and women younger for black men	*
Region	men: some variation women: higher in north	no variation	*	lower in Thames Regions	lower in Thames Regions	no marked variation	some variation	*	*	*

SUMMARY MATRIX (cont.)	rate of conceptions among under 16s	% of deaths due to accidents	death rate from road accidents	casualty rate for road accidents	death rate from fires	casualty rate from fires	death rate from home accidents	non-fatal home injuries	% with smoke alarm fitted
Age	NA	highest among 15–24	highest among 16–19 and 80+	highest among 16–19 and 20–29	highest among 1–4 and 65+	highest among 17–24 and 80+	under 16: highest among 1–4 16+: higher among older	highest among under 5s and 75+ women	highest where HOH 35–44 lowest 75+
Sex	NA	under 65: higher among males 65+: no difference	higher among males	*	higher among men	higher among men	under 75: higher among males 75+: higher among females	no difference	*
Secular Trend	increasing up to 1990	under 15 and over 65: decreasing 15–24: increasing (death rates)	decreasing	decreasing slightly	decreasing	increasing	*	decreasing	increasing
Socio-Economic	*	*	*	*	*	*	*	*	no variation
Economic Activity	*	*	*	*	*	*	*	*	*
Marital Status Household Type	*	*	*	*	*	*	*	*	highest among married with children lowest in single person households
Ethnic Group	*	*	*	*	higher among ethnic minority groups	*	*	*	*
Region	slightly higher in north	SMRs for accidental death: slightly higher in north	SMRs for road accidents: some variation	*	*	*	*	*	lowest in North, Midlands and East higher in Scotland

Notes

1. The figures and tables in this overview are all based on published data. They have been reproduced using the data as they were published except where some figures have been amalgamated. No attempt has been made to standardise the data by age, sex or any other socio-demographic variable. Although some references are made in the text to variation with age and sex within other socio-demographic variables no other form of cross-analysis has been carried out. Thus, it is possible that some apparent variations may, in fact, be due to other confounding factors. This does not invalidate the overall description of the data presented.

2. Information has been presented for England where possible but otherwise, GB or UK figures are used. Data for the component countries of the UK are presented where the data source provides them. Regional tables in the Appendix are based on Regional Health Authorities at the time most of the data reported in the overview were collected (1992/93).

3. The most recent published data available at 31 March 1995 have been used which means that there is some variation in the years referred to.

4. Differences mentioned in the text have been found to be statistically significant at the 95% confidence level.

5. Social class and socio-economic group are based on the occupation of the head of household unless otherwise stated.

6. Further information on any of the surveys, including copies of questionnaires, can be obtained from the NHS Health Survey Advice Centre. This has been set up by the Department of Health and is run by OPCS. Its main aim is to help health authorities get the maximum value from local surveys by advising on ways of improving their quality, and by encouraging the use of standardised methods of collecting data, where appropriate. For details please contact

Eileen Goddard
OPCS Social Survey Division
St Catherines House
10 Kingsway
London WC2B 6JP

Direct line 0171 396 2058
Fax 0171 405 3020

THE VARIATION IN HEALTH RELATED BEHAVIOUR

DIET

HON Targets:

to reduce the average percentage of food energy derived by the population from saturated fatty acids by at least 35% by 2005 (from 17% in 1990 to no more than 11%)

to reduce the average percentage of food energy derived by the population from total fat by at least 12% by 2005 (from about 40% in 1990 to no more than 35%)

The current data source for these targets is the National Food Survey (NFS); a continuous survey which measures household food consumption and expenditure. Data are presented as averages across all people in the household.

The new National Diet and Nutrition Survey programme sponsored jointly by MAFF and DH will cover a different age group approximately every two years and report on the intake of nutrients measured on an individual basis. Following detailed surveys on the diet and health of adults in 1986/7 and on the diets of children between the ages of 6 and 12 months in 1986, the first report in this new series, published in 1995, related to pre-school children. Future surveys will cover elderly people, school age children and adults. The survey of adults will provide data for comparison with the 1986/7 dietary survey of adults.

Intake of nutrients is the result of a combination of different dietary behaviours. Consumption of specific foods or food types can be used as indicators of dietary behaviour but none individually is a proxy for intake of nutrients.

Based on the 1994 COMA report on the Nutritional Aspects of Cardiovascular Diseases, the consumption of five types of food have been selected as indicators of dietary behaviour for inclusion in this overview

milk	usual type of milk consumed
fat spread	usual type used
fruit	reported consumption at least once a day
vegetables/salad	reported consumption at least once a day
bread	reported consumption more than once a day

as measured by the Health Survey for England (1993). Trend data indicating average consumption are available through the NFS.

Secular trends and variation with age and sex Over the past twenty years there was a decrease in the percentage of food energy from saturated fats from 19% to 16%

(GB figures) but the percentage of food energy from total fat remained almost constant (42% in 1972 and 41% in 1993). *Figure D1*

Among people aged 16–64, the percentage of food energy derived from fat and saturated fatty acids was similar across all age groups and for both sexes (GB 1986/7). *Table D1*

This relative stability contrasts strongly with the figures for milk consumption. The average weekly number of pints per person of whole milk decreased from 4.6 in 1972 to 1.6 in 1993. The weekly consumption of low fat milk rose from almost zero to 1.8 pints per person. *Figure D2*

Older people were more likely to report using butter or hard margarine and to have whole fat milk. Women were less likely than men to have whole fat milk but there was no difference between reported use of fat spreads (England 1993). *Figures D3/4*

Consumption of vegetables (especially potatoes) has declined since 1986, while fruit consumption (mainly fruit juice) increased through the 1980s but remained at similar levels between 1991 and 1993. The average consumption of bread declined until 1991 and has since remained at about 27 ounces per person per week which is approximately equivalent to a large loaf. *Figure D5*

68% of women and 64% of men said they ate vegetables or salad at least daily. The proportion who said they ate fruit at least daily was considerably higher for women than men (54% and 43%). The majority of both men and women reported eating bread every day but a greater proportion of men reported eating bread more than once a day (39% compared with 30%). *Table D2*

Socio-economic variation The percentage of food energy derived from fat and from saturated fatty acids showed no significant variation with social class. People in non-manual households were less likely to use whole milk but there was no variation in the use of different types of fat spread. *Figures D6/7*

The highest reported frequency of eating vegetables, salad and fruit was among those in social classes I and II and the lowest among those in IV and V. For example, 78% of women in social classes I or II reported eating vegetables or salad at least daily compared with 57% of women in classes IV or V. Men in manual workers households were slightly more likely to report eating bread more than once a day. *Figure D8*

Employment status There was no variation with employment status in the percentage of food energy derived from fat and saturated fatty acids. *Table D3*

Household type Total fat provided slightly higher proportions of food energy for people living in households of 3 or more adults. *Table D4*

Geographical variation There was no significant regional variation with respect to fat intake. In terms of dietary behaviour, the Health Survey for England reported that people in the north were less likely to eat fruit, vegetables or salad but more likely to eat bread more than once a day. The usual type of fat spread and milk also varied with region for both men and women (for example the proportion of men who reported using butter or hard margarine ranged from 30% in North East

Thames to 16% in Trent). Consumption of fruit and vegetables was lower in Scotland than England. *Figure D9, Regional Tables in appendix*

References and notes

MAFF. National Food Survey 1993, London HMSO 1994. GB. A continuous survey which collects details of all food brought into the home in one week. For an individual household, the quantity of food thus obtained for consumption, or estimates of nutrient intake derived from it, may differ from actual consumption because of changes in household stocks during the week and because of wastage. The data are presented averaged across all people.

MAFF. National Food Survey 1990, London HMSO 1991. GB. This report gives trend data.

OPCS. Health Survey for England 1993, London HMSO 1995. Age 16+

OPCS. The Dietary and Nutritional Survey of British Adults (1986/7), London HMSO 1990 Age 16–64

Mills A and Tyler H. Food and Nutrient Intakes of British Infants Aged 6–12 Months, London HMSO 1992

DH. Report on Health and Social Subjects 46, Nutritional Aspects of Cardiovascular Diseases Report of the Cardiovascular Review Group. Committee on Medical Aspects of Food Policy. London HMSO 1994

Table D1 *Percentage of food energy from saturated fatty acids and total fat*

	Percentage of food energy from				**Base Area, Year, Sample**	
	Saturates		**Total fat**		GB 1986/7	
	Men	**Women**	**Men**	**Women**	16–64	
Age						
16–24	16	16	40	40	*214*	*189*
25–34	16	17	41	41	*254*	*253*
35–49	16	17	40	40	*346*	*385*
50–64	17	18	40	40	*273*	*283*
16–64	16	17	40	40	*1,087*	*1,110*

Source: OPCS The Dietary and Nutritional Survey of British Adults

Table D2 *Regular consumption of fruit, vegetables and bread among men and women*

	Proportion eating Vegetables/salad at least daily	Fruit at least daily	Bread more than once a day	Base Area, Year, Sample
				England 93
Men	64	43	39	approx[1] 7,550
Women	68	54	30	approx 8,850

[1]Bases exclude informants whose frequency of eating each food was not known
Source: OPCS Health Survey for England

Table D3 *Percentage of food energy from saturated fatty acids and total fat*

	Percentage of food energy from				Base Area, Year, Sample	
	Saturates		Total fat			
	Men	Women	Men	Women	GB 1986/7	
Employment Status					16–64	
Working	17	17	41	40	*875*	*670*
Unemployed	16	17	39	40	*99*	*57*
Econ. inactive	16	17	39	40	*111*	*373*

Source: OPCS The Dietary and Nutritional Survey of British Adults

Table D4 *Percentage of food energy from saturated fatty acids and total fat*

Household composition		Percentage of food energy from saturates	total fat	Base Area, Year, Sample
Adults	Children			
1	0	16	41	
1	1+	16	41	
2	0	16	41	
2	1	16	41	GB 1993
2	2	16	41	All ages
2	3	16	40	
2	4+	15	40	8,043 Hhlds
3	0	16	42	
3+	1–2	16	41	
3+	3+	15	43	
4+	0	17	43	

Source: MAFF National Food Survey

Figure D1: Percentage of Food Energy from Fat
All Ages Great Britain 1972–1993

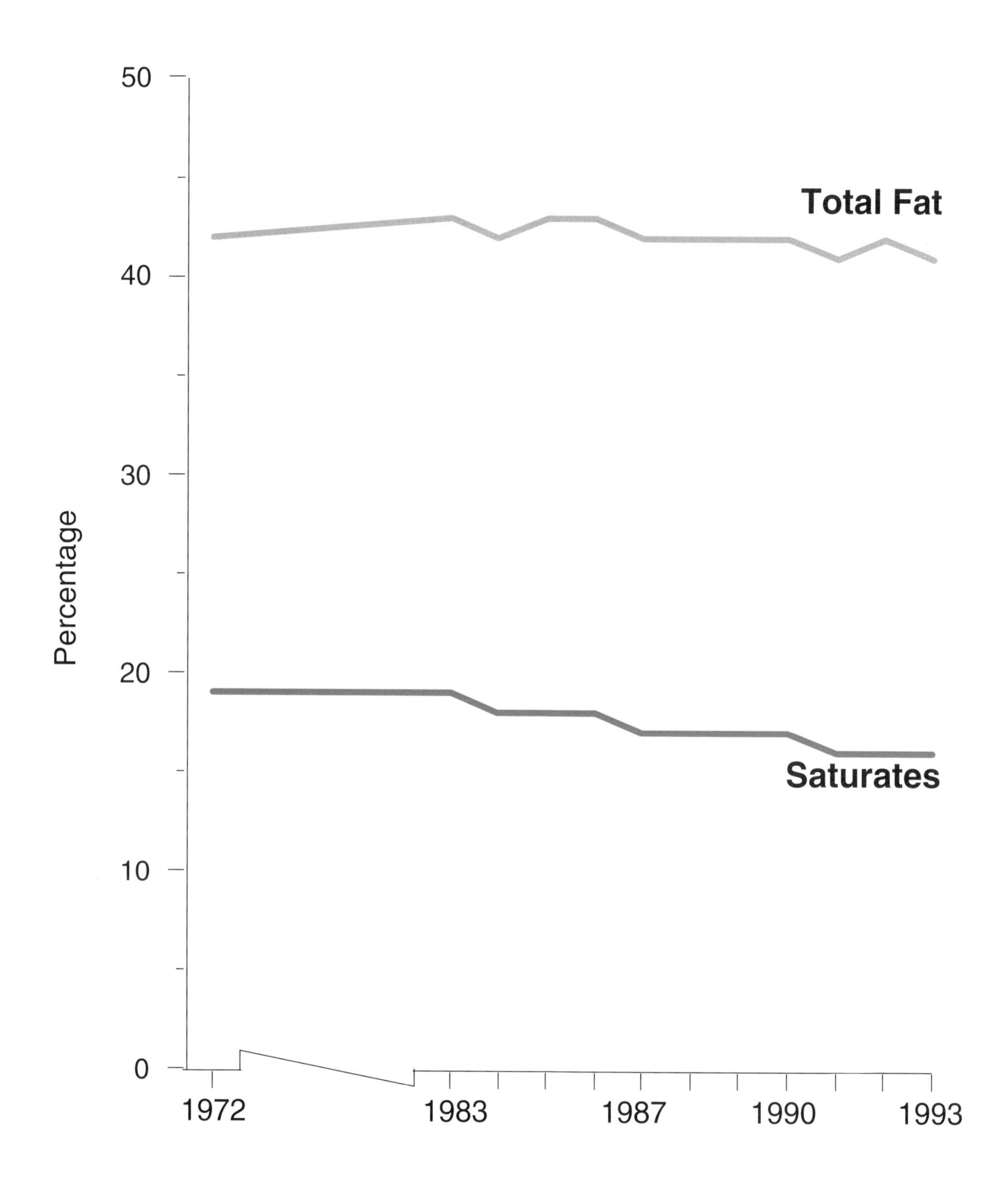

Source: MAFF National Food Survey

Figure D2: Average† Consumption of Milk
All Ages Great Britain 1972–1993

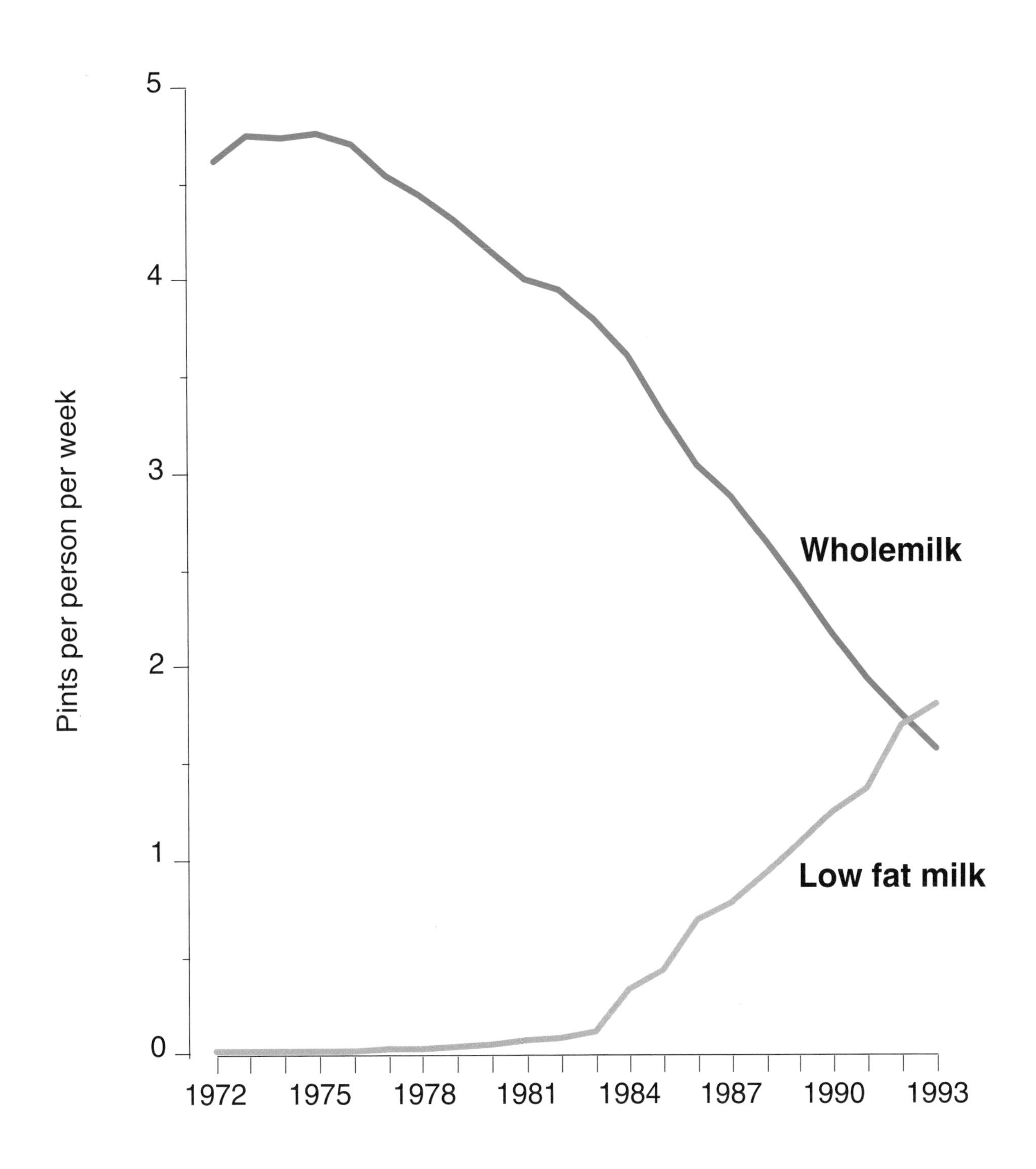

† Average per person calculated from household data
Source: MAFF National Food Survey

Figure D3: **Usual Type of Fat Spread Used**
by Age & Sex England 1993

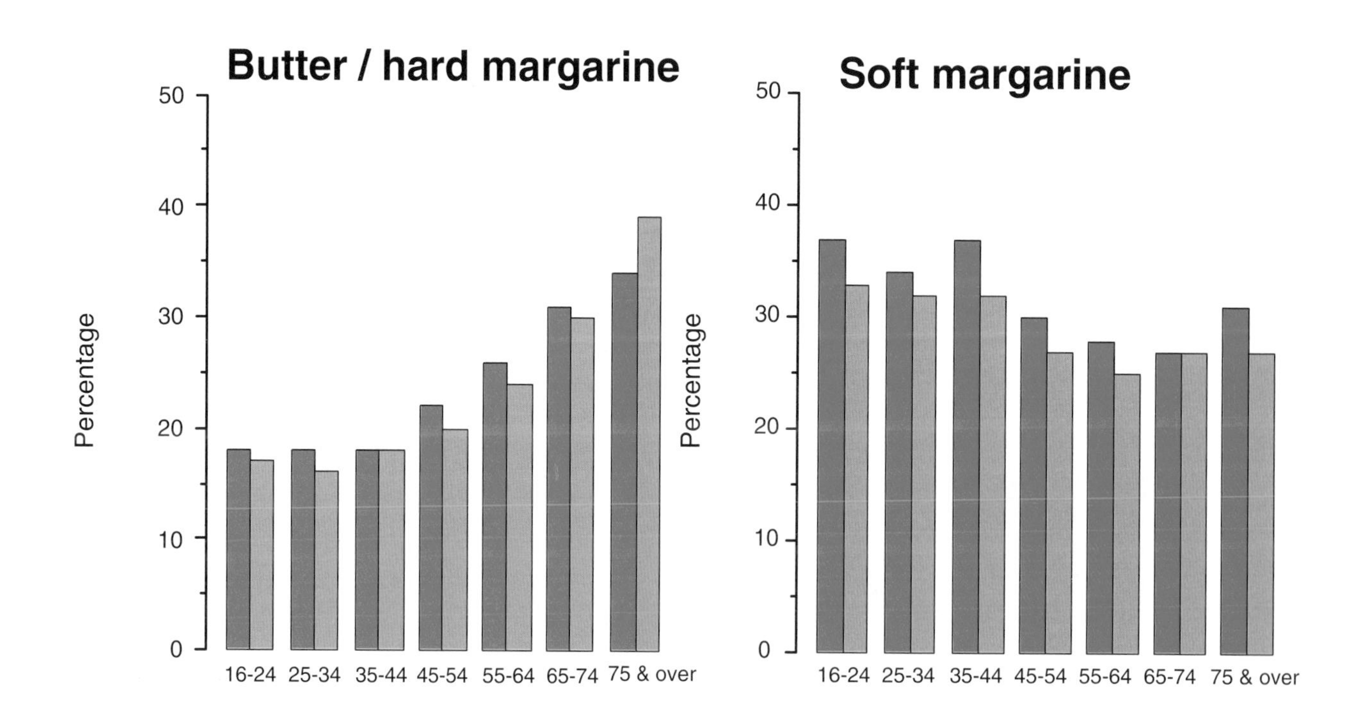

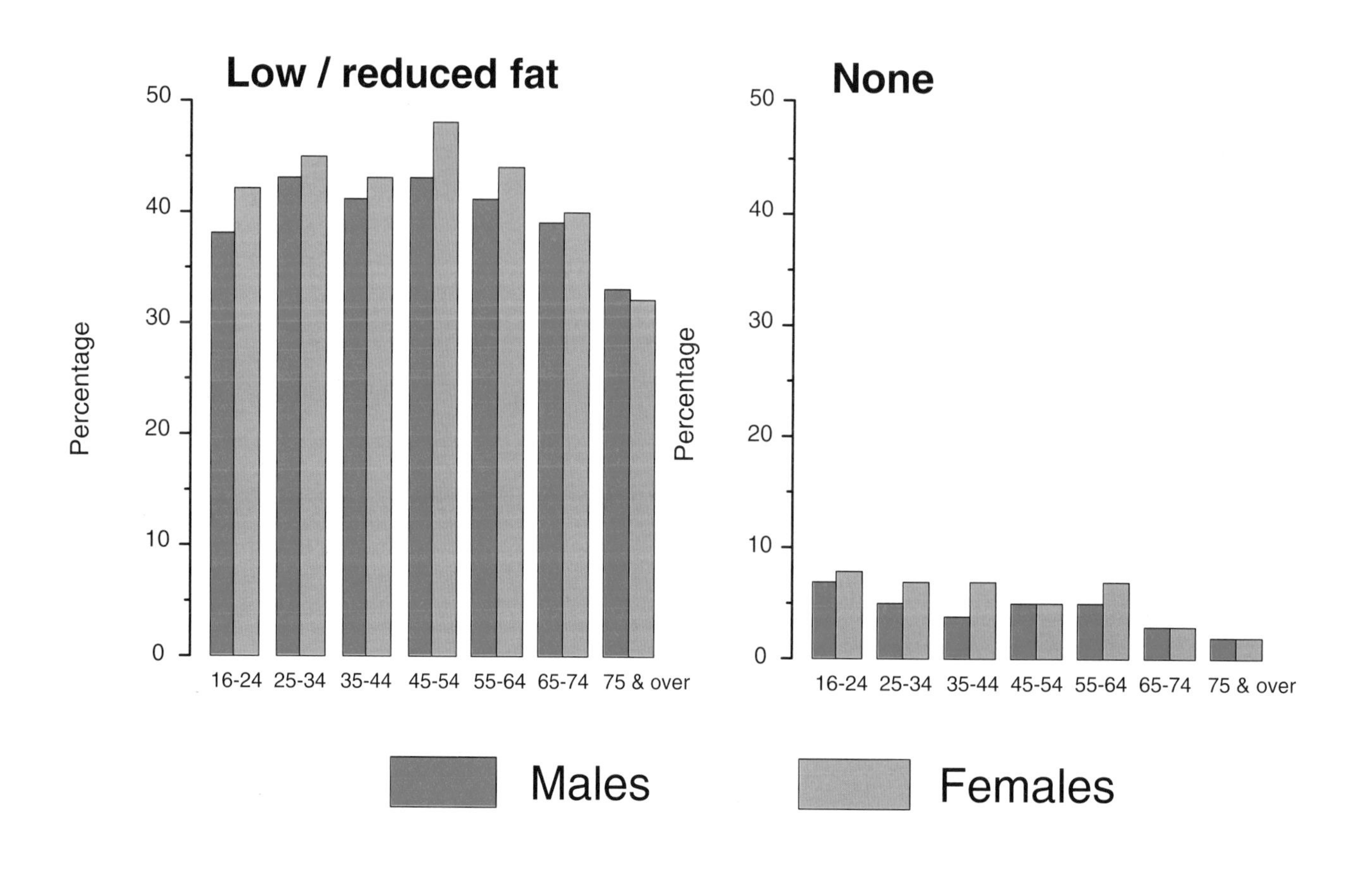

Source: OPCS Health Survey for England

Figure D4: **Usual Type of Milk Consumed**
by Age & Sex England 1993

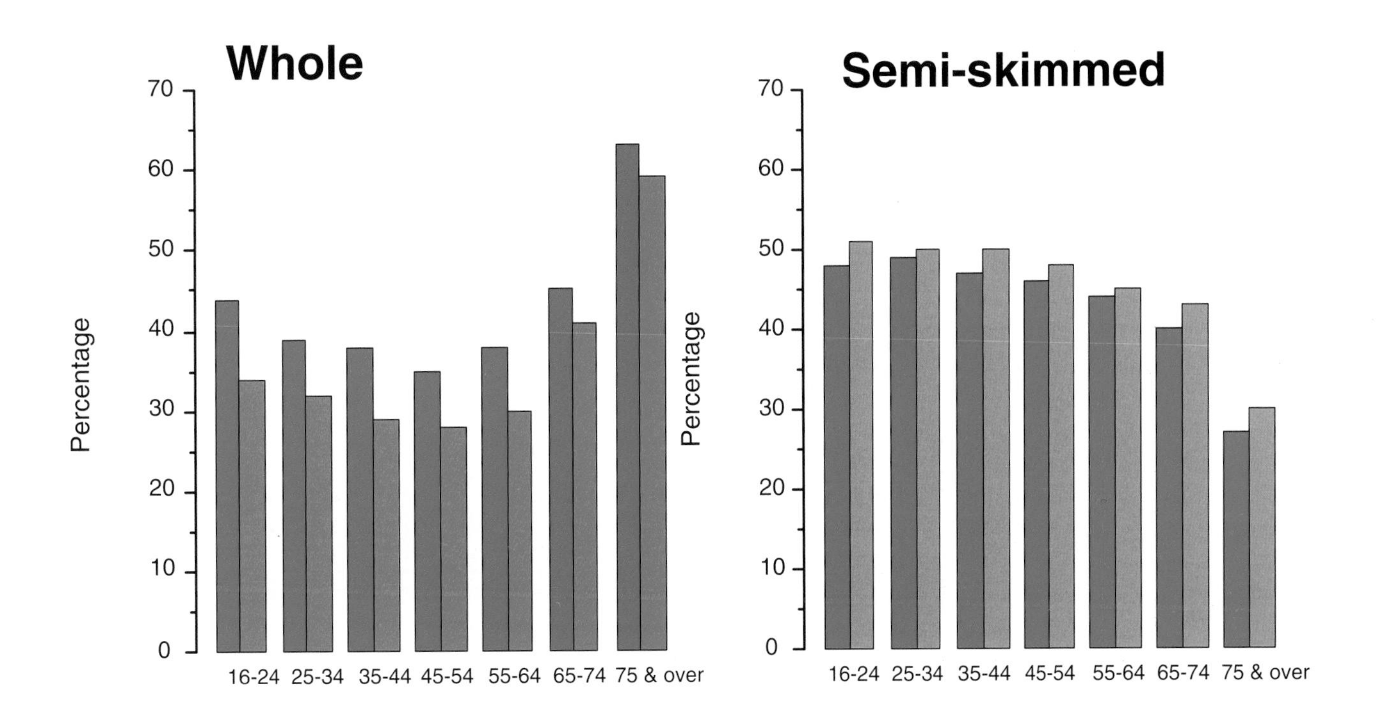

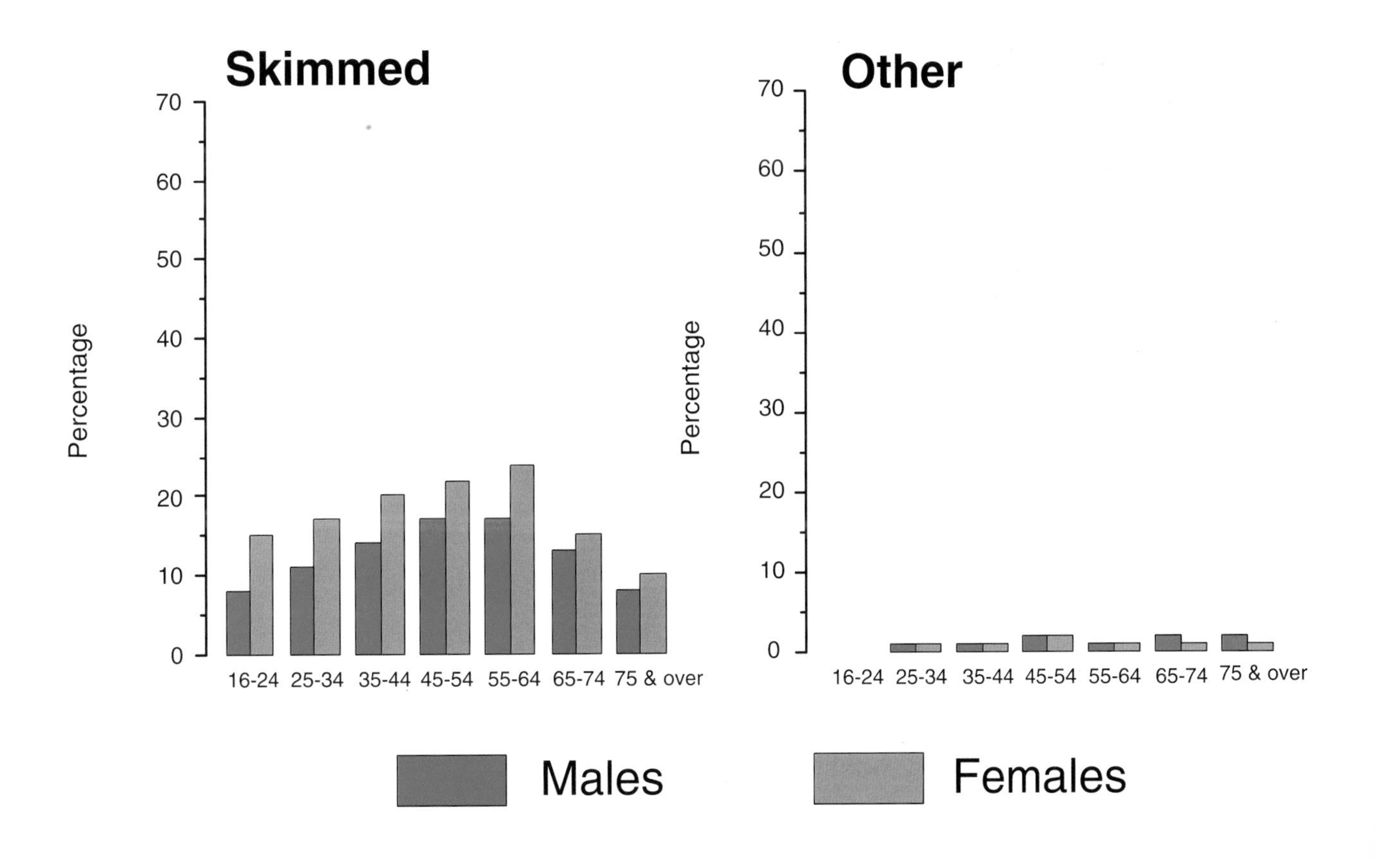

Source: OPCS Health Survey for England

Figure D5: Average† Consumption of Selected Foods
All Ages Great Britain 1972–1993

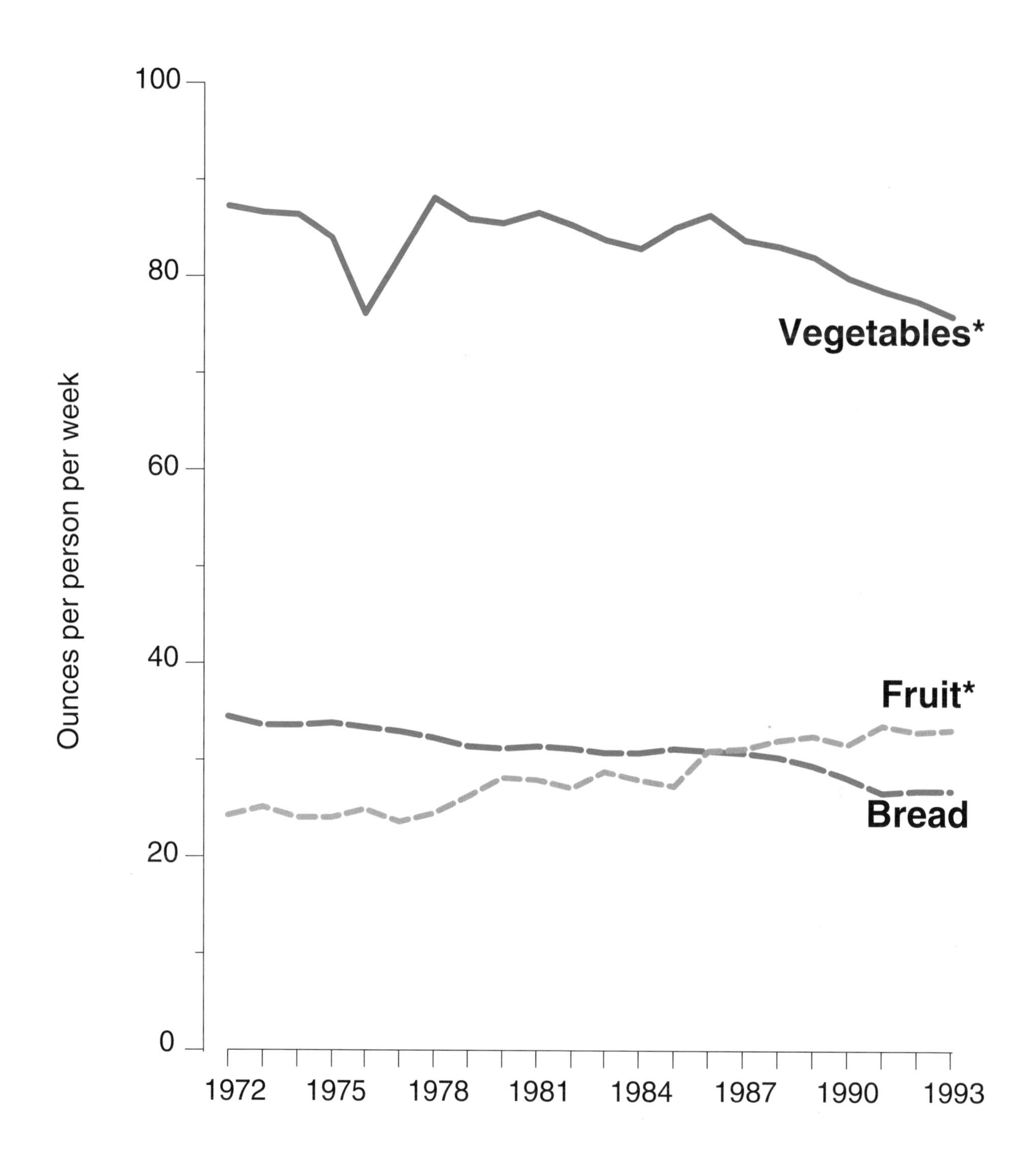

* Vegetables: fresh, frozen and other
Fruit: fresh and other, includes fruit juice
† Average per person calculated from household data
Source: MAFF National Food Survey

Figure D6: Percentage of Food energy from Saturated fatty acids and total fat
by Sex & Social class Age 16–64 Great Britain 1986/87

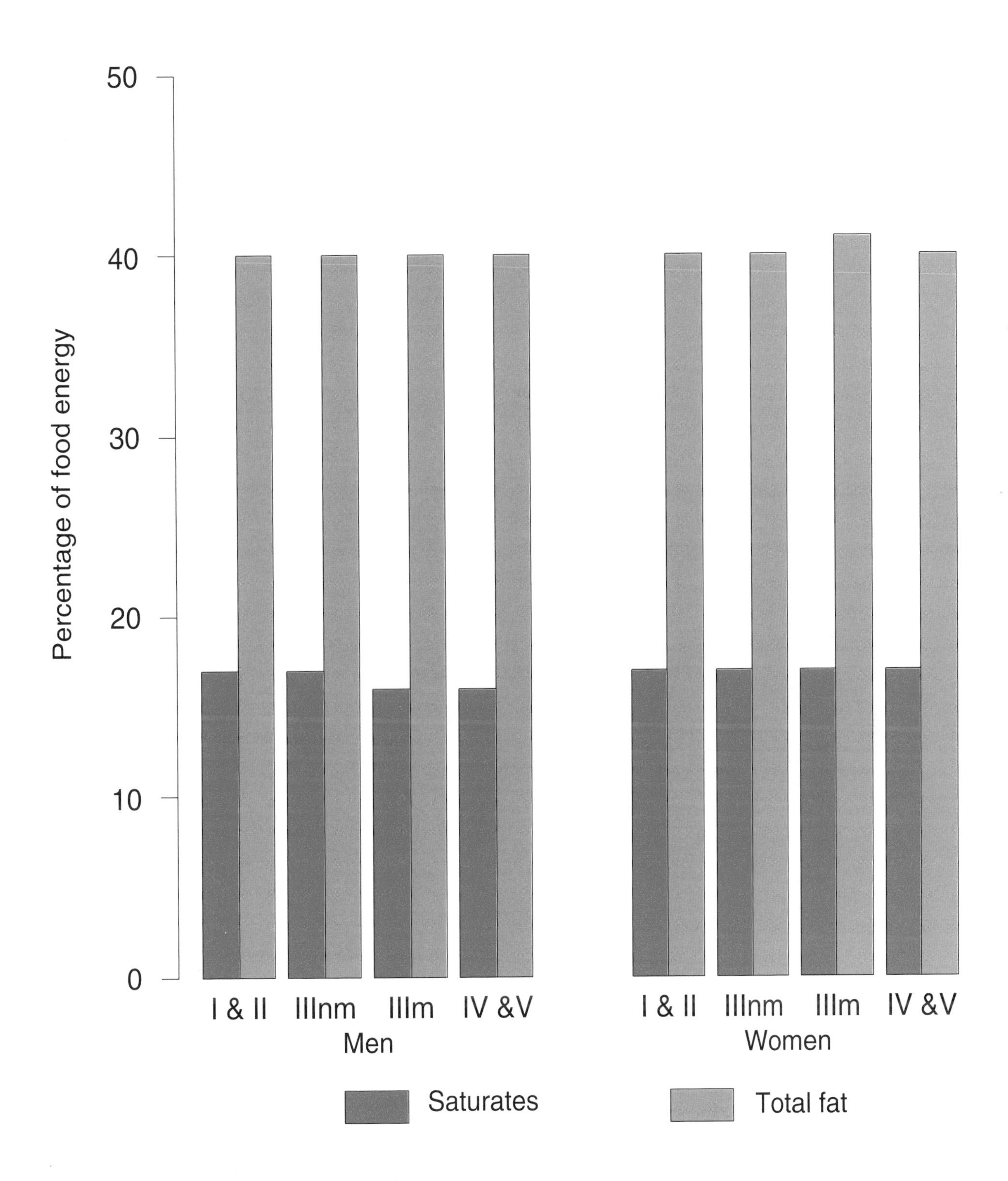

Source: OPCS The Dietary and Nutritional Survey Of British Adults

Figure D7: Usual type of Milk Consumed
by Sex & Social Class Age 16+ England 1993

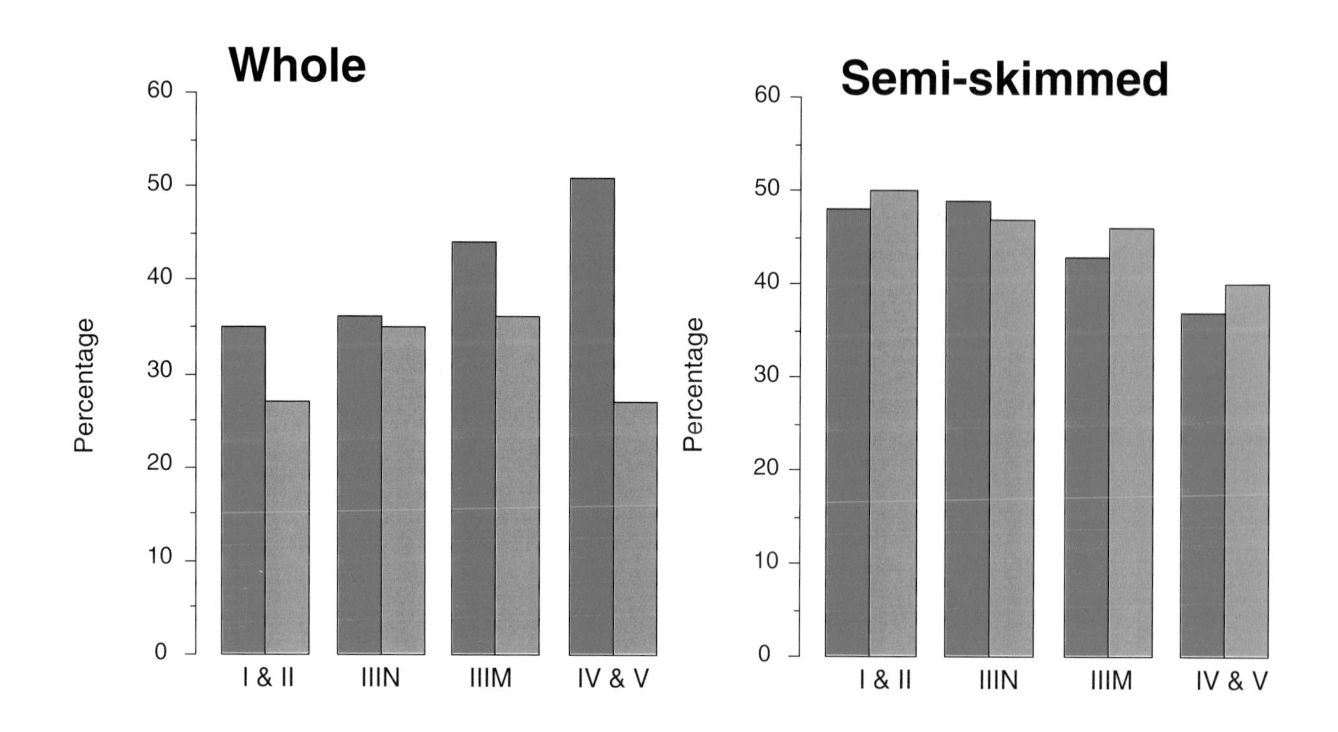

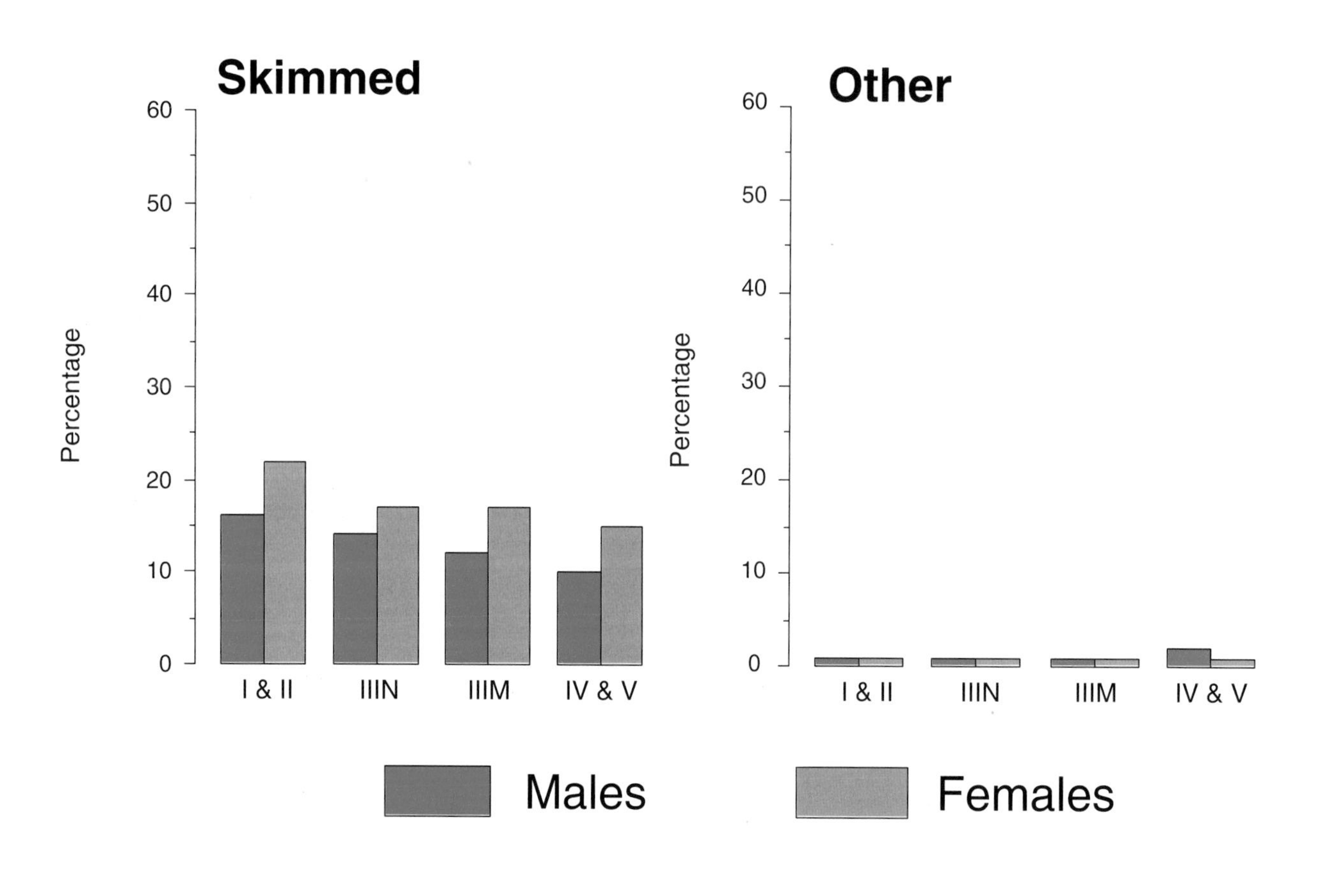

Excludes those who do not drink milk or do not have a usual type
* Social class of head of household (as defined by occupation)
Source: OPCS Health Survey for England

Figure D8: Frequency of Eating Certain Food
by Social Class & Sex Age 16+ England 1993

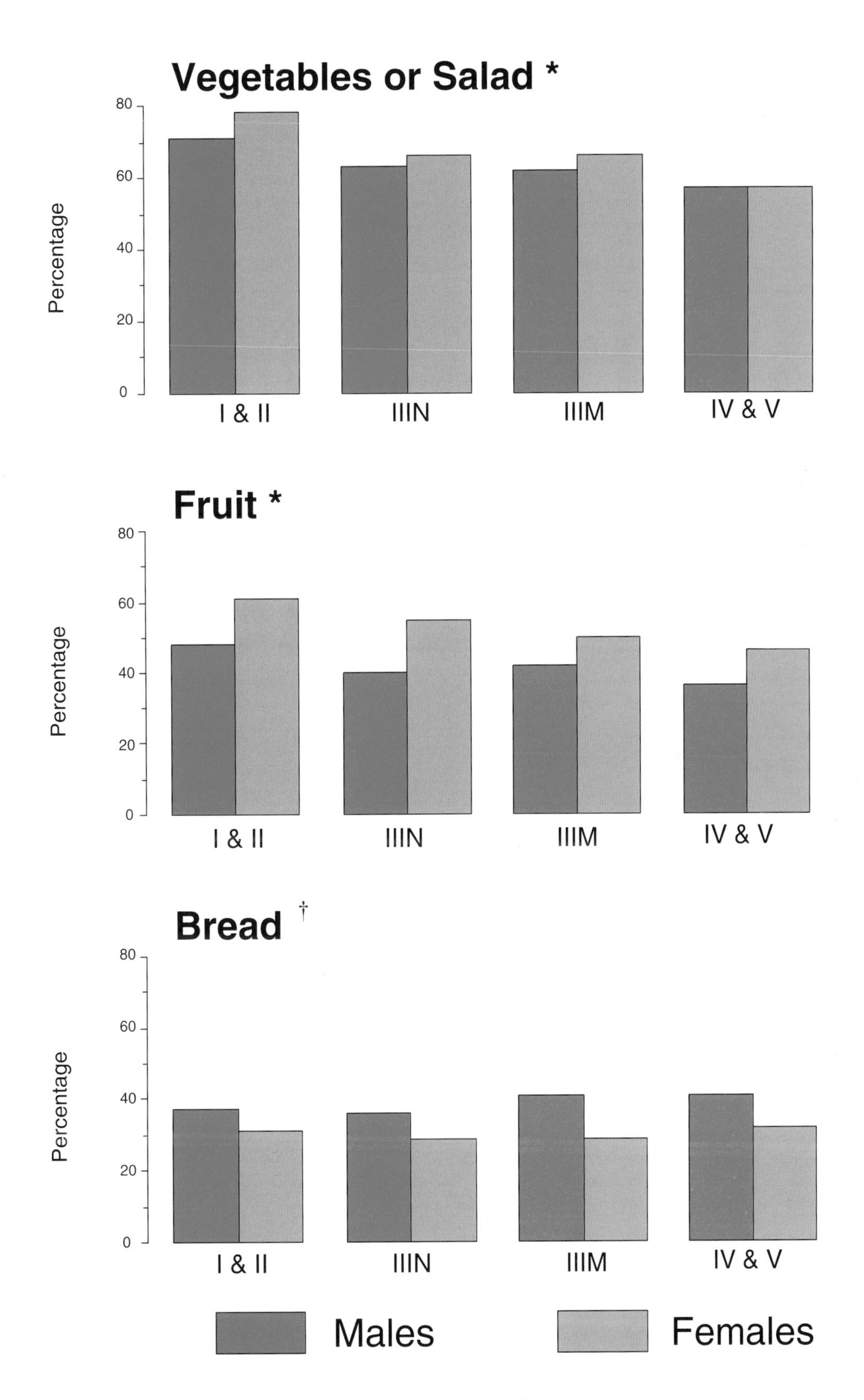

Social class of head of household (as defined by occupation)
* Eaten once a day or more
† Eaten more than once a day
Source: OPCS Health Survey for England

Figure D9: Percentage of Food energy from Saturated fatty acids and total fat
by Region All Ages Great Britain 1993

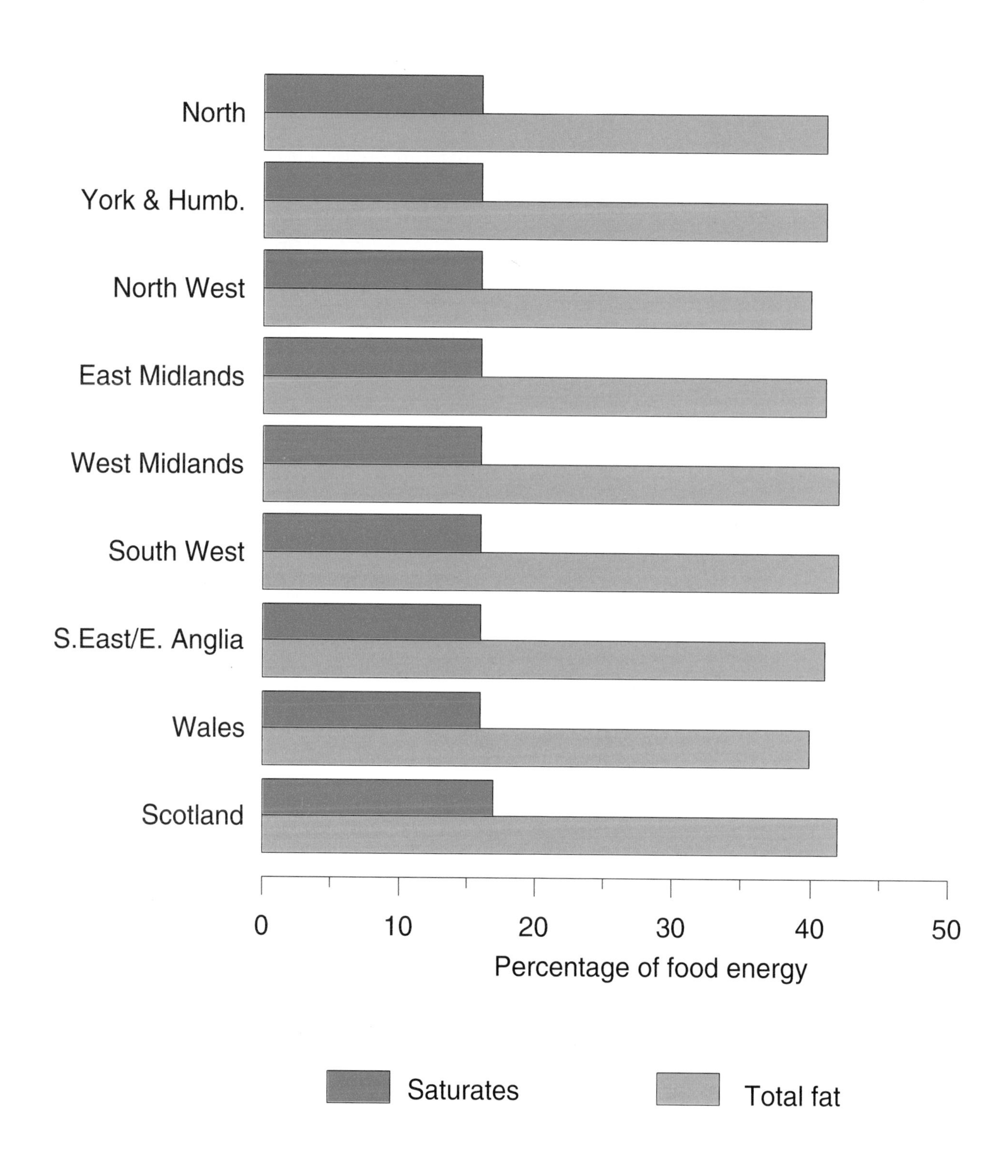

Source: MAFF National Food Survey

ALCOHOL CONSUMPTION

HON Targets:

to reduce the proportion of men drinking more than 21 units of alcohol per week from 28% in 1990 to 18% by 2005 and the proportion of women drinking more than 14 units of alcohol per week from 11% in 1990 to 7% by 2005

The Health of the Nation states that drinking less than 21 units of alcohol per week for men and 14 units per week for women is unlikely to damage health. Sustained alcohol consumption in excess of these levels is likely to lead to increasing health risks. Consumption in excess of 50 units per week for men and 35 units for women is considered to be a dangerous level of drinking.

The target for alcohol consumption refers to a specific behaviour. The baseline percentages come from the General Household Survey and are calculated from reported frequency of drinking together with usual amount drunk. Thus the data do not give precise measures of intake but serve to identify broad groups with different levels of alcohol consumption. The target figures refer to people aged 18 and over.

As a further indicator, deaths and injuries from road accidents involving alcohol have also been included in this overview.

Secular trends and variation with age and sex In 1992 in Great Britain, 27% of men and 11% of women aged 18 and over drank above the recommended sensible levels of 21 and 14 units a week respectively. In England, 26% of men, and 12% of women, drank above these levels. (The recommended levels have since been revised; the data shown refer to the recommended levels at the time of data collection.) Six per cent of men and 2% of women in Great Britain drank above the level considered to be definitely dangerous to health and analysis by age showed this figure was 11% for men aged 18 to 24. *Figure AL1*

The proportion of men with an alcohol consumption above the sensible level has remained steady since 1986, but there is an indication of an increase among men aged 45 or more. The proportion of women drinking above a sensible level increased from 9% in 1984 to 11% in 1992. First figures from the OPCS Survey of Psychiatric Morbidity indicate that the overall rate of alcohol dependence was 47 per thousand (or 5%) in the past year (1993–4; GB; aged 16–64). (See notes for definition of dependence.) *Figures AL1–2*

Drinking above the recommended sensible level was most common among men and women aged 18–24 (38% and 18% respectively). *Figure AL2*

Among 15 year olds in England in 1992, 36% of boys and 20% of girls said they drank at least once a week. *Figure AL3*

In 1993, 5% of all road accident injuries were in accidents where the driver had an alcohol level above the legal limit, and 14% of all fatalities occurred in alcohol related accidents. *Table AL1*

The number of casualties (including pedestrians) in road accidents involving drivers with illegal alcohol levels declined from an estimated 18,800 in 1982 to 10,840 in 1993. Data were not available to distinguish between types of road users. *Figure AL4*

Socio-economic variation Among people aged 16 and over, women in the non-manual groups were more likely to drink above the recommended sensible level than those in the manual groups. The variation among men was less clear, but more of those in the employers/managers group and in the unskilled manual group were drinking above the sensible level (29% and 28% respectively above the sensible level compared, for example, with 22% of those in the semi-skilled and junior non-manual groups). *Figure AL5*

Employment status There was very little difference between those in work and the unemployed in the proportions who were drinking above the recommended sensible level. The smaller proportions among the economically inactive for both men and women are in part due to the older age profile of this group. *Figure AL6*

Marital status Men who were divorced, separated or single were more likely to drink above a sensible level than married men while those who were widowed were least likely. Among women the differences were not so large but those who were widowed were also the least likely to drink above a sensible level. Some of this variation is due to the strong relationship between marital status and age. *Figure AL7*

Geographical variation Men in the northern regions were, in general, more likely than men elsewhere to exceed the recommended sensible level: 32% of men in the North Western region drank more than 21 units per week compared with 18% of men in the North East Thames region. Among the women there was also some variation with region but there was no evidence of a north-south trend. *Figure AL8*

Among people aged 16 and over, there was little difference in alcohol consumption between men in Scotland, Wales and England (26%, 28% and 26% over the sensible level) but a smaller proportion of women in Scotland drank over the sensible level (8% compared with 12% in England and 11% in Wales).

References and notes

Alcohol consumption is described in the Figures as

> 'Heavy' (22–50 units per week for men and 15–35 units per week for women)
>
> 'Very heavy' (51 units per week and over for men and 36 units per week and over for women).

These divisions are based on the HON target for alcohol and the accompanying notes in the White Paper. Both the General Household Survey and the Health

Survey for England employ three groups 'fairly high' and 'high' which together are equivalent to 'heavy', and 'very high' which is equivalent to 'very heavy' in this review.

The OPCS Surveys of Psychiatric Morbidity define alcohol dependence as 3 or more positive responses to a list of 12 statements covering loss of control, symptomatic behaviour, and binge drinking. The statements are listed in full in Bulletin No. 1 of the Survey.

OPCS. General Household Survey 1992, London HMSO 1994 (Series GHS; no. 23) GB. Questions on alcohol consumption were asked of age 18+ up to 1987. From 1988 16–17 year olds were given self-completion questionnaires. It is suggested the overall proportions may be underestimates because

i) quantities of alcohol drunk at home are underestimated

ii) heavy drinkers may be under-represented in the sample because of non-response. People in institutions and those living rough are excluded.

DoT. Road Accidents Great Britain 1993 The Casualty Report London HMSO 1994. The figures presented on casualties in alcohol related road accidents are based on estimates. A full description of this procedure is given in the report.

Figures for drinking among secondary school children come from OPCS Smoking among secondary school children in 1992, London HMSO 1993.

OPCS. Surveys of Psychiatric Morbidity in Great Britain Bulletin No. 1, OPCS 1994

Figure AL1: Alcohol Consumption

Age 18+ Great Britain 1984, 1988 & 1992

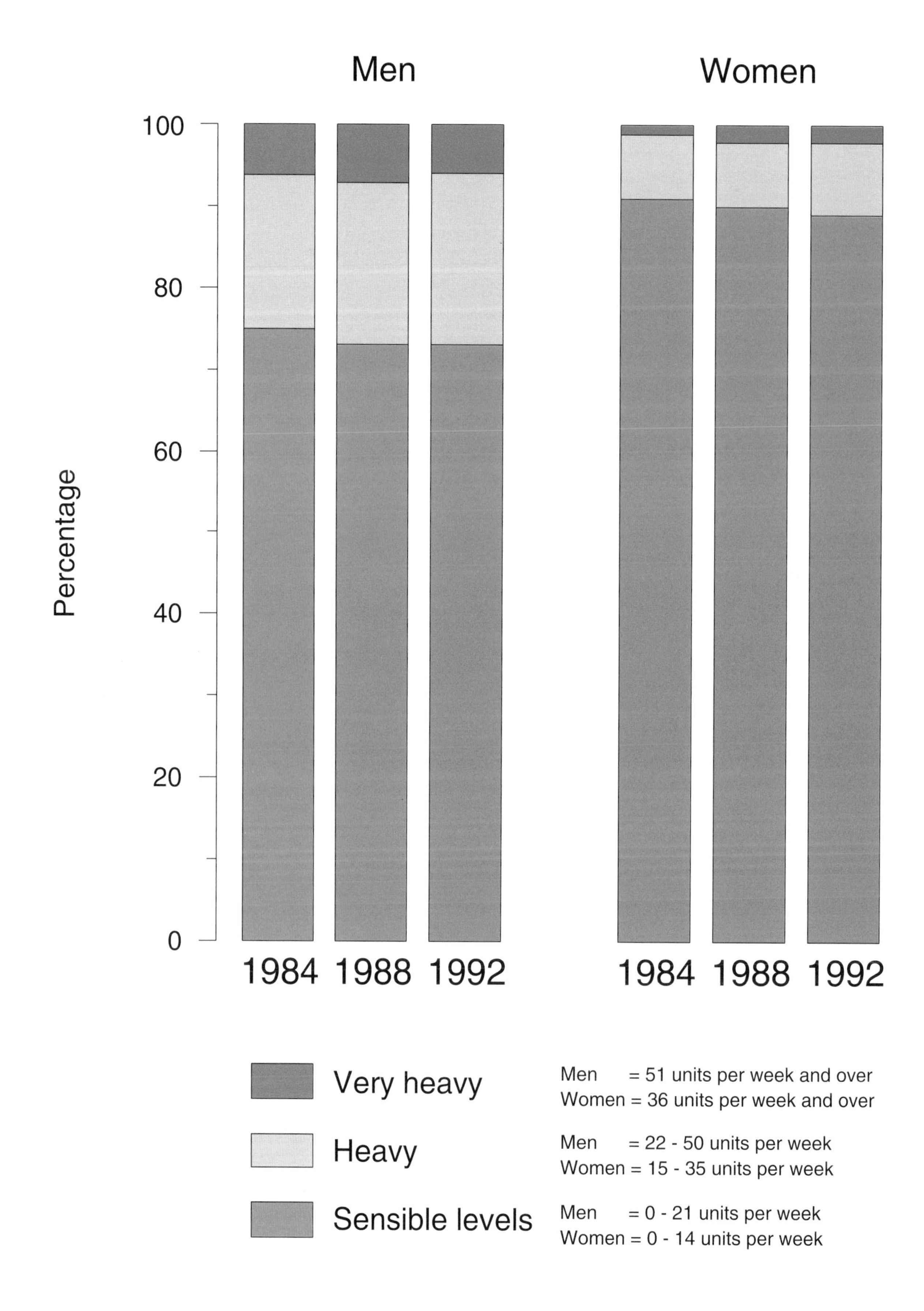

Source: OPCS General Household Survey

Figure AL2: Alcohol Consumption above Sensible Level†
by Age Great Britain 1984–1992

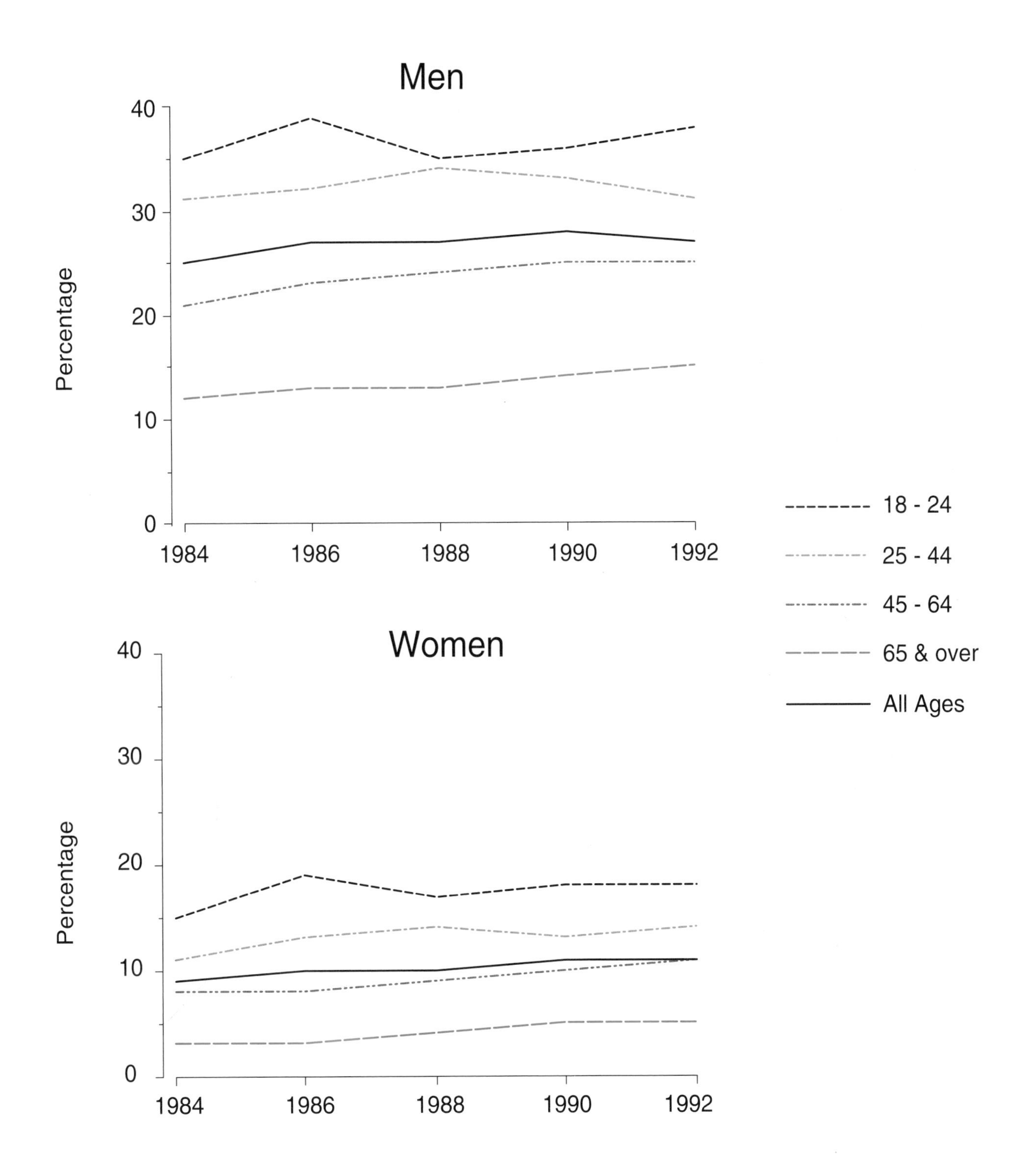

† More than 21 units per week exceeds the sensible level for men
More than 14 units per week exceeds the sensible level for women
Source: OPCS General Household Survey

Figure AL3: Usual Drinking Frequency
by Age & Sex England 1992

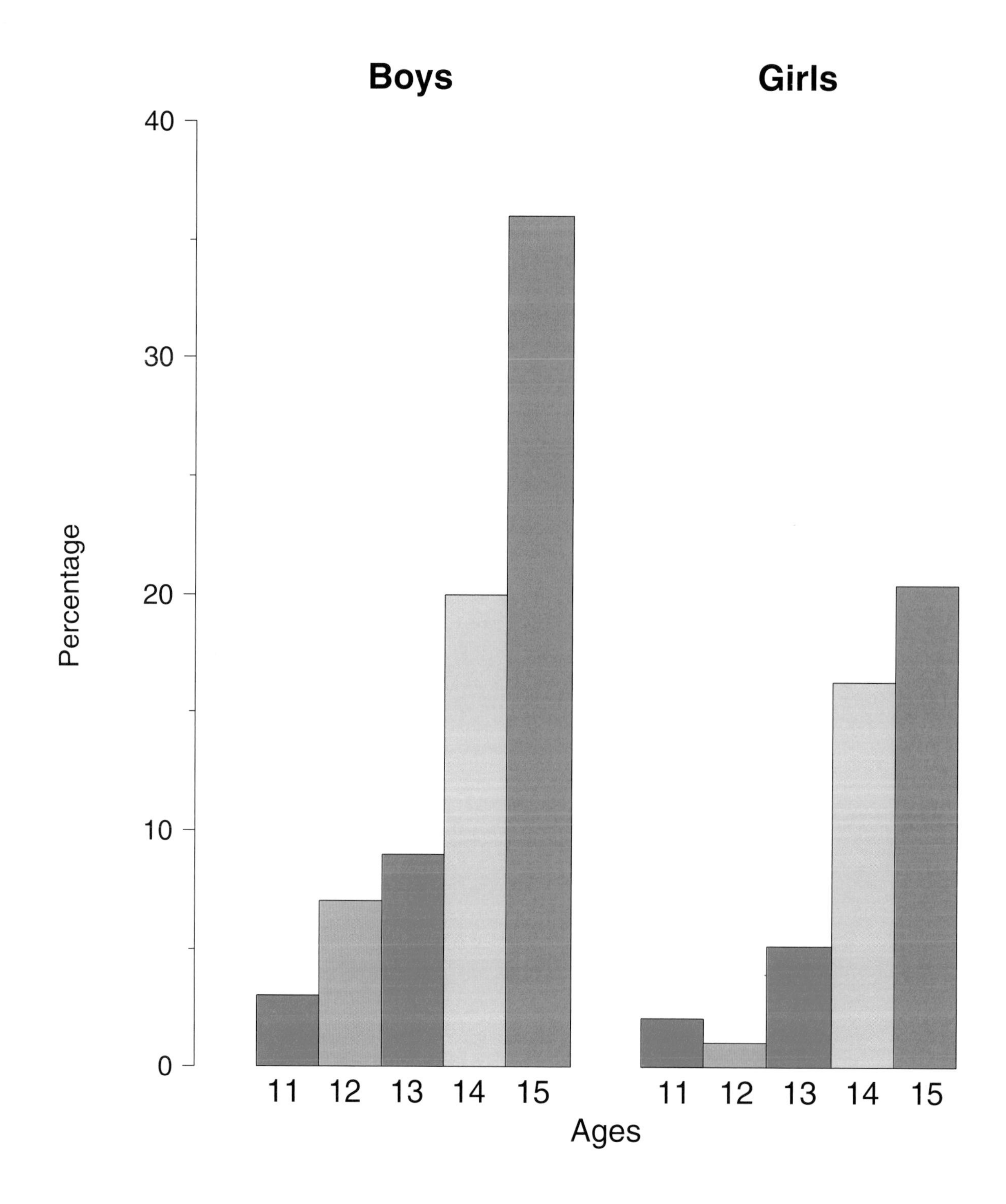

Secondary school children drinking at least once a week
Source: OPCS Smoking among Secondary School Children

Table AL1 *Proportion of casualties involved in alcohol-related accidents*

All casualties	Killed	Seriously injured	Slightly injured
5%	14%	6%	5%

Base = all casualties in road accidents
Source: DoT. Road Accidents Great Britain 1993 The Casualty Report

Figure AL4: Road Accidents and Casualties Involving drivers with Illegal Alcohol Levels
All Ages Great Britain 1982–1993

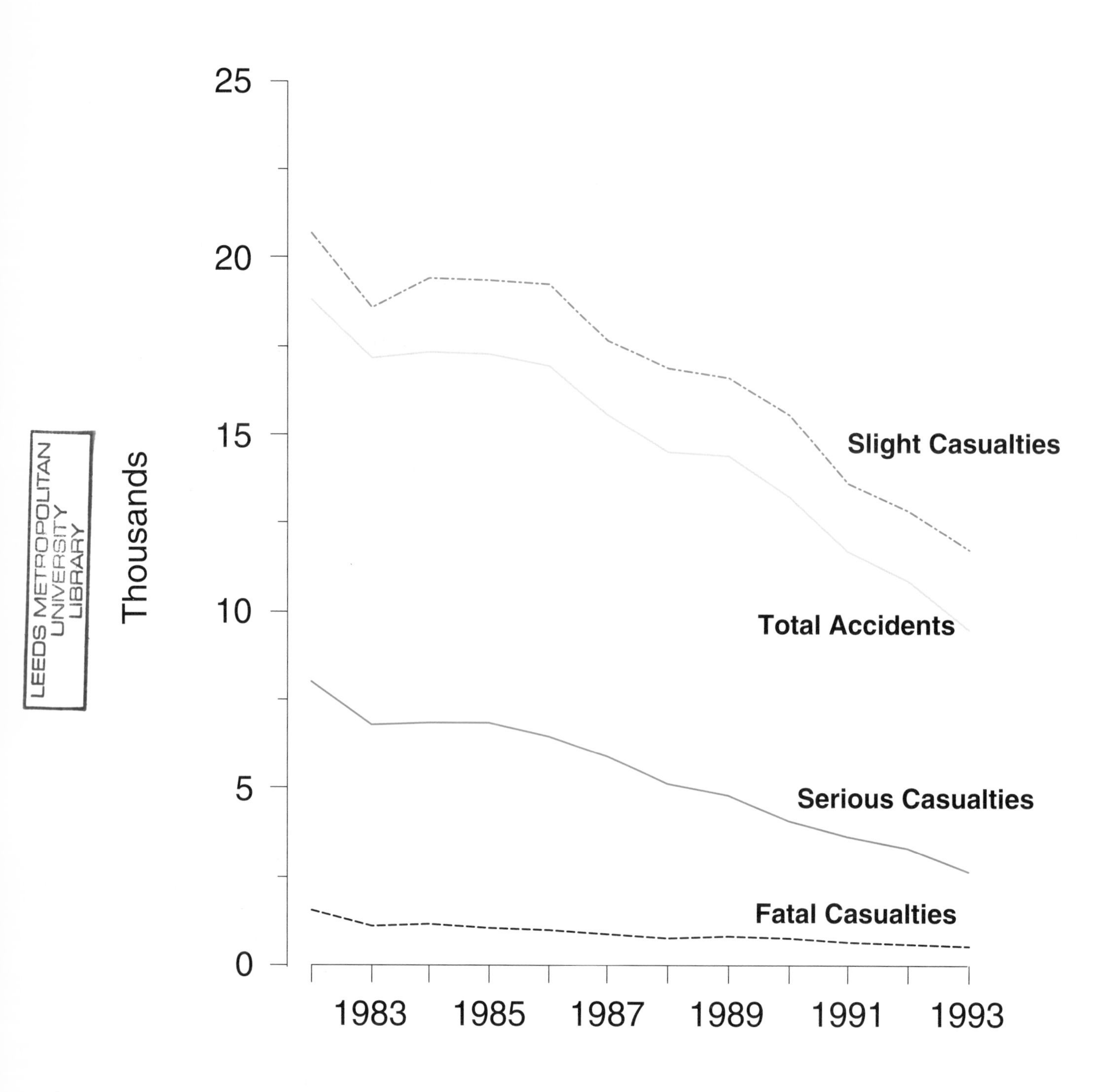

The number of casualties is greater than the total number of accidents as there may be more than one casualty involved with a single accident.
Source: DoT Road Accidents GB 1993 – The Casualty Report

Figure AL5: Alcohol Consumption above Sensible Level
by Socio-Economic Group, Aged 16+ Great Britain 1992

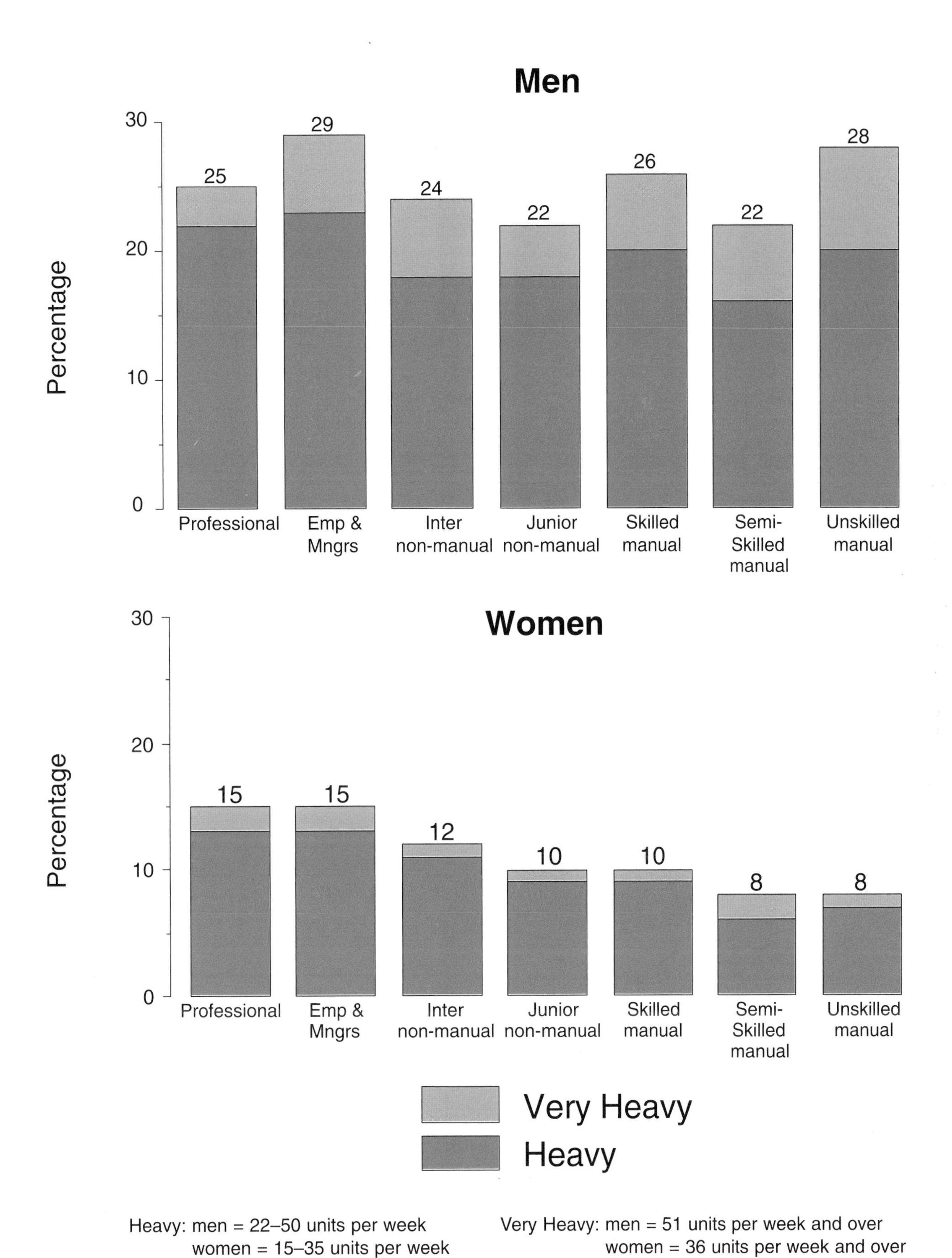

Heavy: men = 22–50 units per week
women = 15–35 units per week

Very Heavy: men = 51 units per week and over
women = 36 units per week and over

Source: OPCS General Household Survey

Figure AL6: Alcohol Consumption above Sensible Level
by Economic Activity Status, Aged 16–64 Great Britain 1992

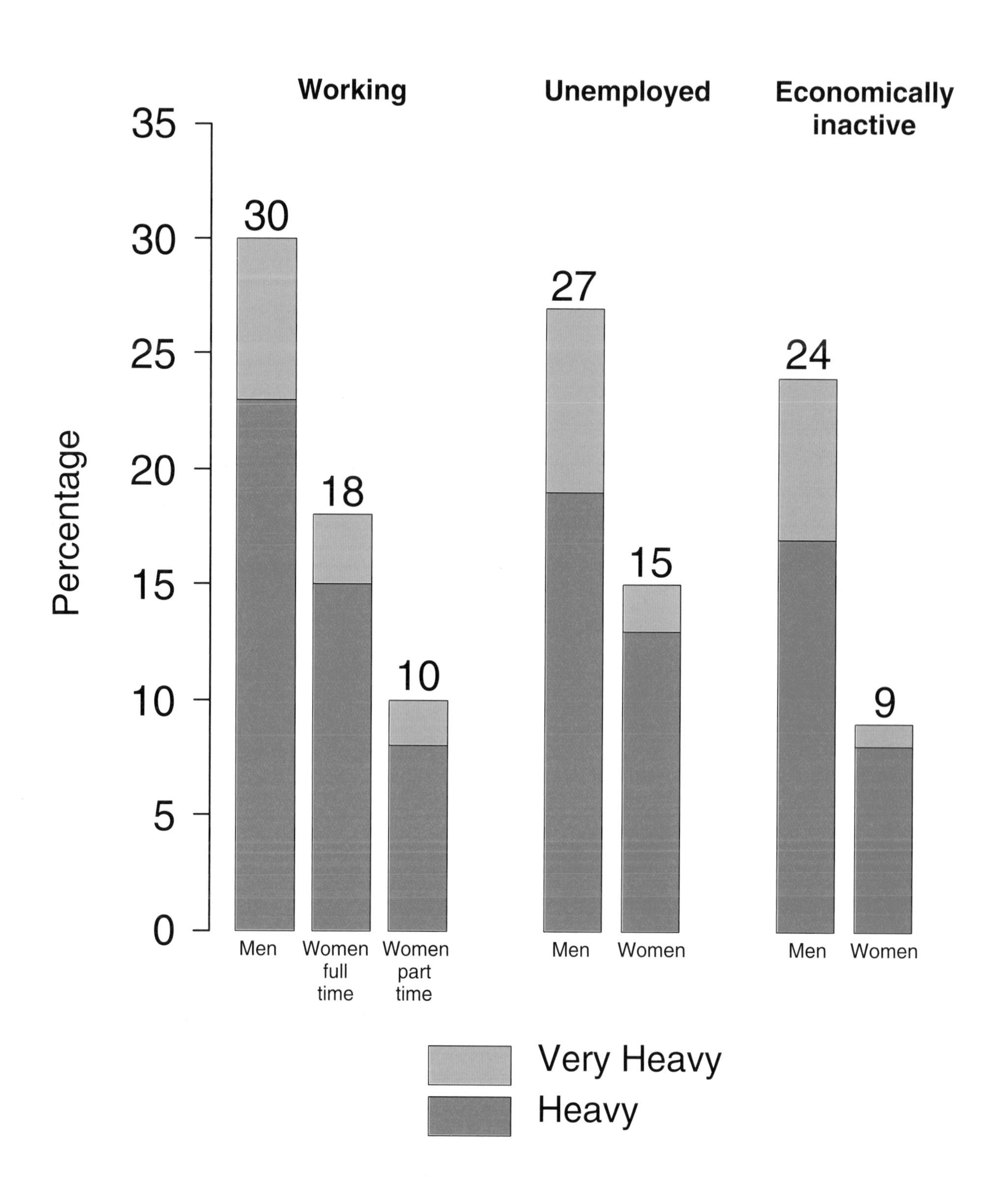

Heavy: men = 22–50 units per week
women = 15–35 units per week

Very Heavy: men = 51 units per week and over
women = 36 units per week and over

Source: OPCS General Household Survey

Figure AL7: Alcohol Consumption above Sensible Level
by Marital Status, Aged 16+ Great Britain 1992

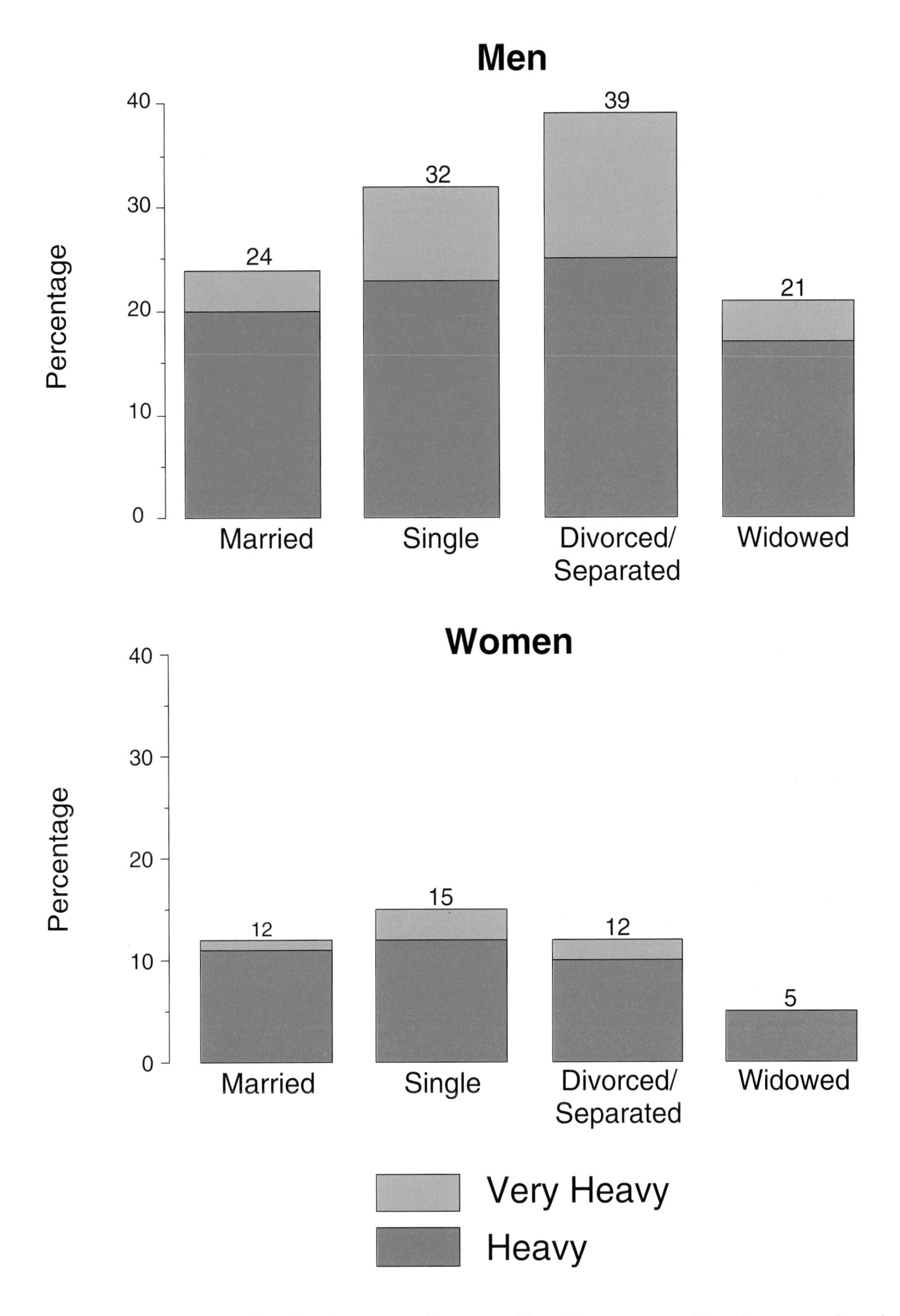

Heavy: men = 22–50 units per week
women = 15–35 units per week

Very Heavy: men = 51 units per week and over
women = 36 units per week and over

Source: OPCS General Household Survey

Figure AL8: Alcohol Consumption Above Sensible Level
by RHA, Age 16+ England 1992

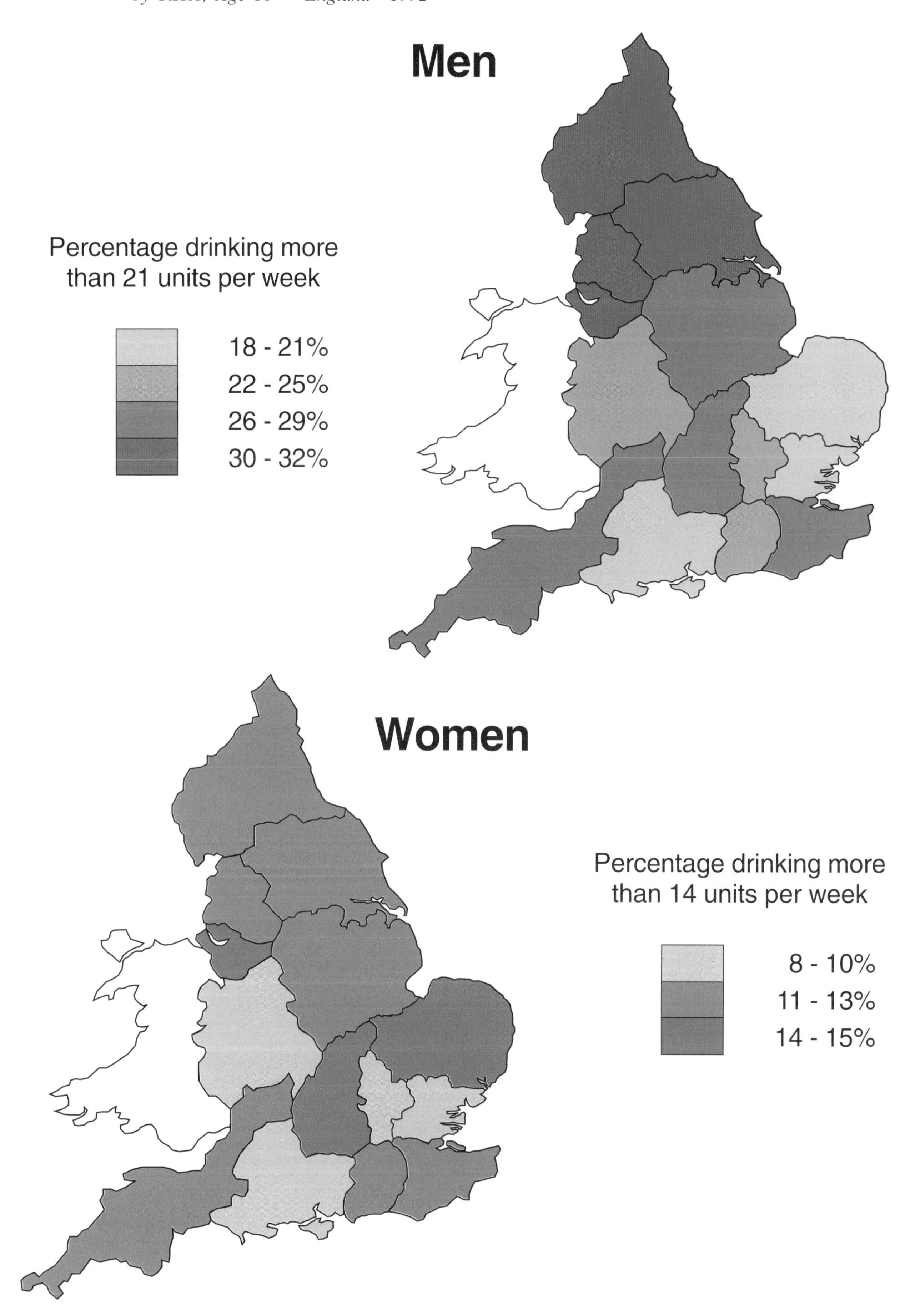

Source: OPCS General Household Survey

PHYSICAL ACTIVITY

Until 1990, no national data regarding overall levels of physical activity within the general population were available. The General Household Survey provides data on leisure time activities but the Allied Dunbar National Fitness Survey (ADNFS) provided the first comprehensive data set on all aspects of physical activity, at work, at home and at leisure. The survey also included a physical appraisal to assess fitness levels. To add to the data set a second interview-only survey was conducted in 1991 – the HEA National Survey of Activity and Health (HEANSAH).

The Health Survey for England 1991–93 included a module on physical activity, using questions and analysis methods similar to the ADNFS.

Three indicators of physical activity are used in this overview

participation in vigorous activity at least 3 times a week for 20 minutes per occasion (eg squash, running, vigorous swimming and some occupations)

participation in at least moderate intensity activity 5 times a week for 30 minutes per occasion (eg brisk walking, digging, spring cleaning, less vigorous swimming, some occupations)

no participation in at least moderate activity lasting 30 minutes or more (sedentary)

The inclusion of both vigorous and moderate intensity activity in these indicators reflect the current scientific opinion that while it is vigorous activity which is associated with the maximum benefit for cardio-respiratory fitness, higher volumes of moderate activity should bring long term health benefits.

Secular trends and variation with age and sex Participation in both vigorous and moderate physical activity declined with age. A greater proportion of men than women were physically active particularly in vigorous intensity activity. In 1993, 10% of men and 4% of women were active at a vigorous intensity three or more times a week for at least 20 minutes per occasion. Participation in such activity was highest among 16–24 year old men (26%). *Figure PA1*

There were similar variations in activity of at least moderate intensity although the proportions participating at this level were considerably higher. In 1990–91, 36% of men and 22% of women had taken part in at least moderate activity 5 or more times a week for 30 minutes per occasion. Over half of the youngest men had participated at this level (52%) but only a quarter of the youngest women had done so (26%). Women in the 25–44 age group were more active than the youngest women.

Over half (55% and 54%) of men and women aged 65–74 were sedentary (active less than once a week at the appropriate level) and as many as 25% of the youngest women were in this category. *Figure PA2*

Comparison of the ADNFS figures and figures from the Health Survey in 1991–1993 showed no evidence of a change in participation in physical activity.

Socio-economic variation A greater proportion of men in households headed by a manual worker were regularly active at both moderate and vigorous intensity levels. These variations mainly reflect the contribution made by occupational activity to overall levels. A smaller but equivalent difference was found between the proportions of women who took regular activity of a moderate intensity or above. The proportions of women regularly active at the vigorous level were too small to show significant differences.

There was less variation in the proportion of sedentary people within each social class group and the differences did not reflect those found for regular activity. Men in the manual group were slightly more likely to be sedentary than those in the non-manual group (33% in group V compared with 27% in group I). Among women, those in classes III non-manual and V were the most likely to be sedentary.

Figures PA3–4

Employment status The contribution made by occupation to regular levels of physical activity among men can once again be seen in the comparison of activity levels of working and unemployed men. For women, there was no such difference.

The proportion of sedentary men was considerably higher among the unemployed (34% compared with 22% of men who were working). A similar gradient was seen among the women although the difference was not statistically significant. The higher proportions of sedentary people among the economically inactive partly reflected the older age profile of this group. *Figure PA5*

Geographical variation There was little regional variation in levels of physical activity. *Figure PA6*

Ethnic Group When asked in the HEA survey of Black and Minority Ethnic Communities whether they did anything to keep or improve their health, 30% of African-Caribbeans, 29% of Indians, 24% of Pakistanis and 20% of Bangladeshis mentioned participation in sports activities. This compared with 39% of the UK population as a whole. More detailed activity data were collected and will be available towards the end of 1995.

References and notes

The Sports Council and Health Education Authority. Allied Dunbar National Fitness Survey – main findings, Sports Council London 1992
Age 16+ England The main analysis was limited to people aged 16-74

OPCS. Health Survey for England 1993, London HMSO 1995
Age 16+ England

Killoran A, Fentem P, Casperson C, (eds) Moving On. International perspectives on promoting physical activity, HEA London 1995. This report contains analysis of the merged data set from the ADNFS and HEANSAH surveys. More data will be found in HEA. Health Update – Physical Activity, HEA London 1995

HEA Black and Minority Ethnic Groups in England, HEA 1994 Age 16–74

Figure PA1: Regular Participation† in vigorous Physical Activity
by Age & Sex England 1993

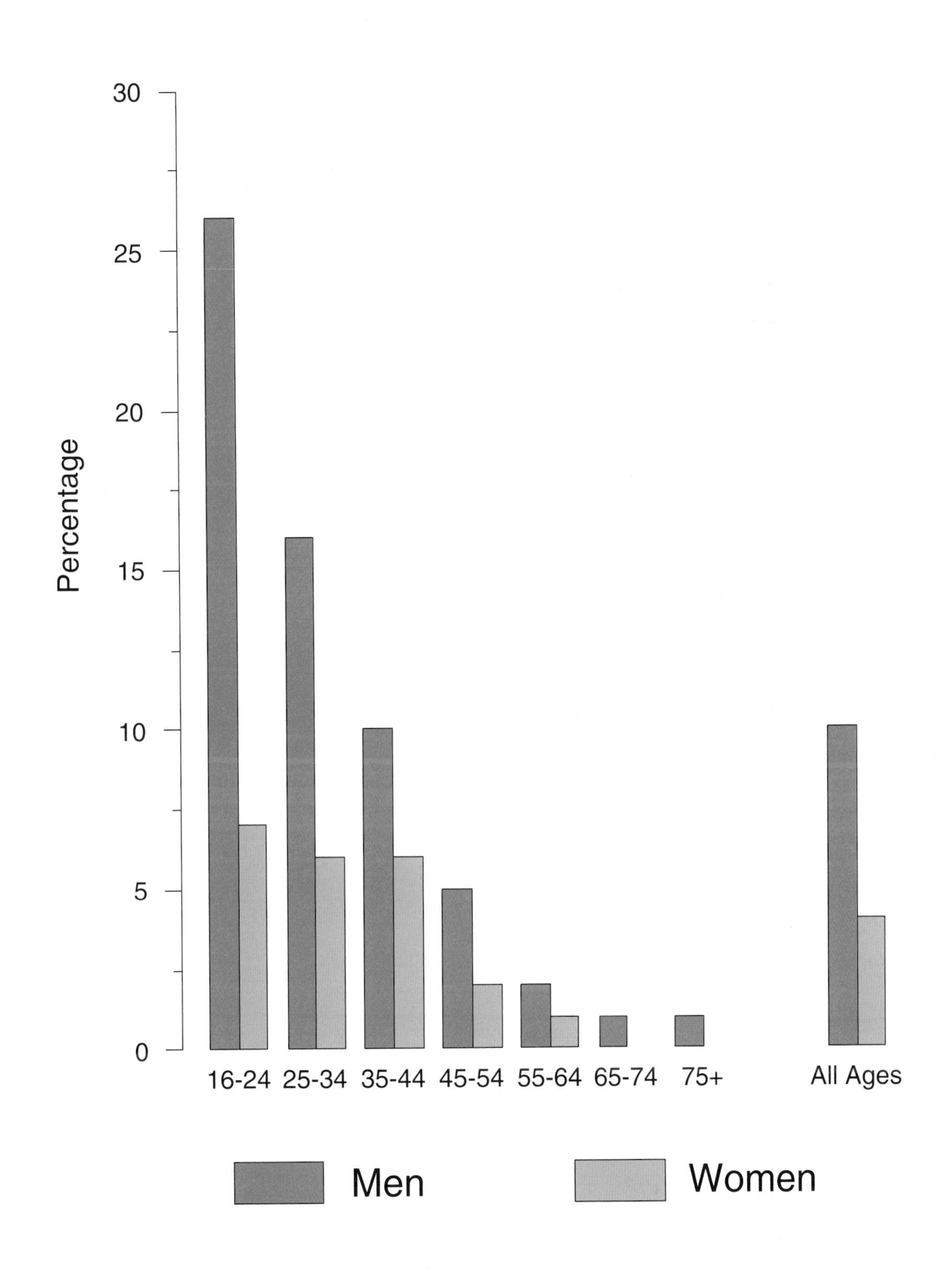

† Regular Participation: 20 minutes at least 3 times a week
Source: OPCS Health Survey for England

Figure PA2: Participation in Physical Activity of at least moderate intensity
by Age & Sex England 1990/91

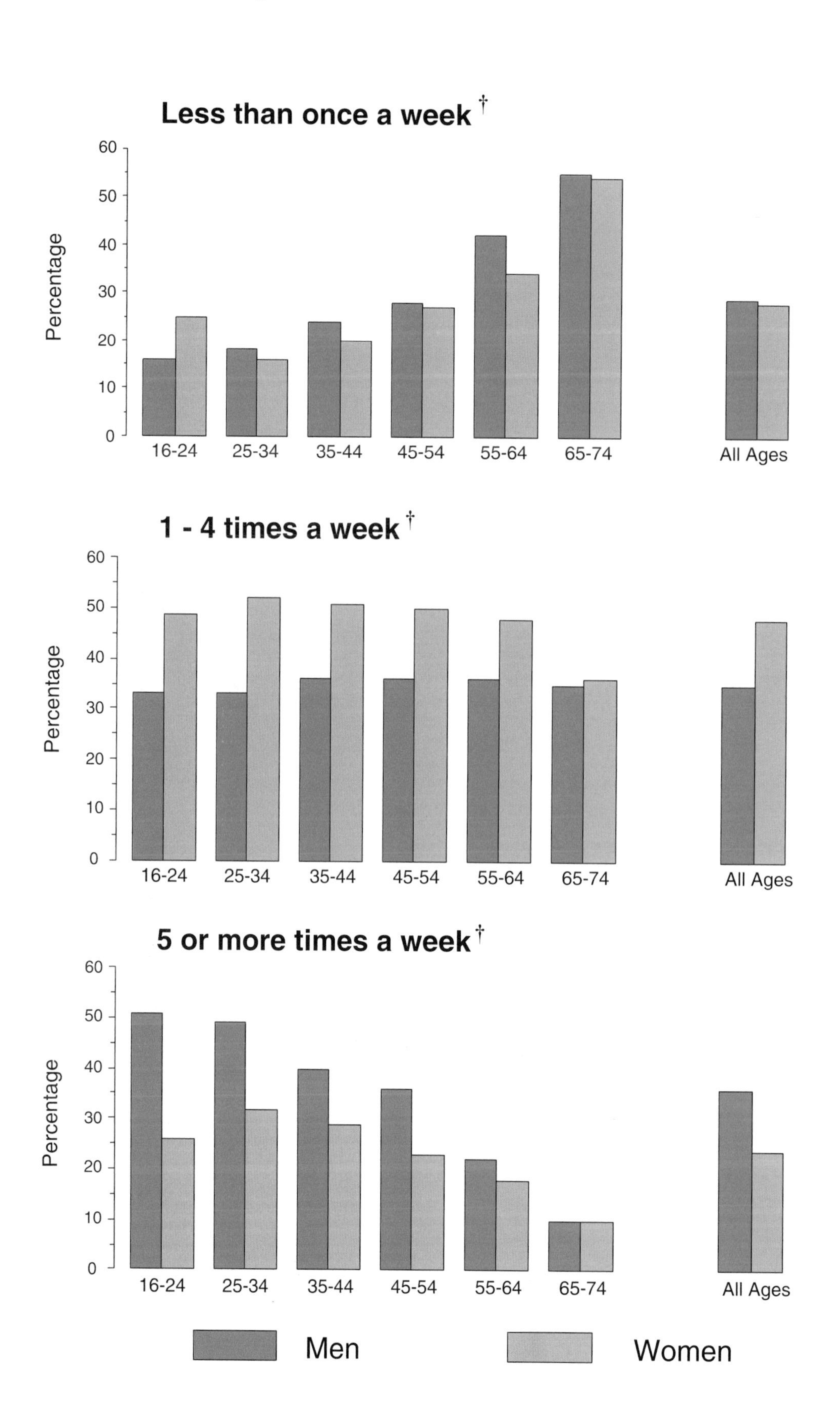

† 30 minutes per occasion

Source: HEA/Sports Council,
Allied Dunbar National Fitness Survey,
HEA National Survey of Activity & Health

Figure PA3: Regular Participation† in Vigorous Physical Activity
by Social Class, Age 16–74 England 1990*

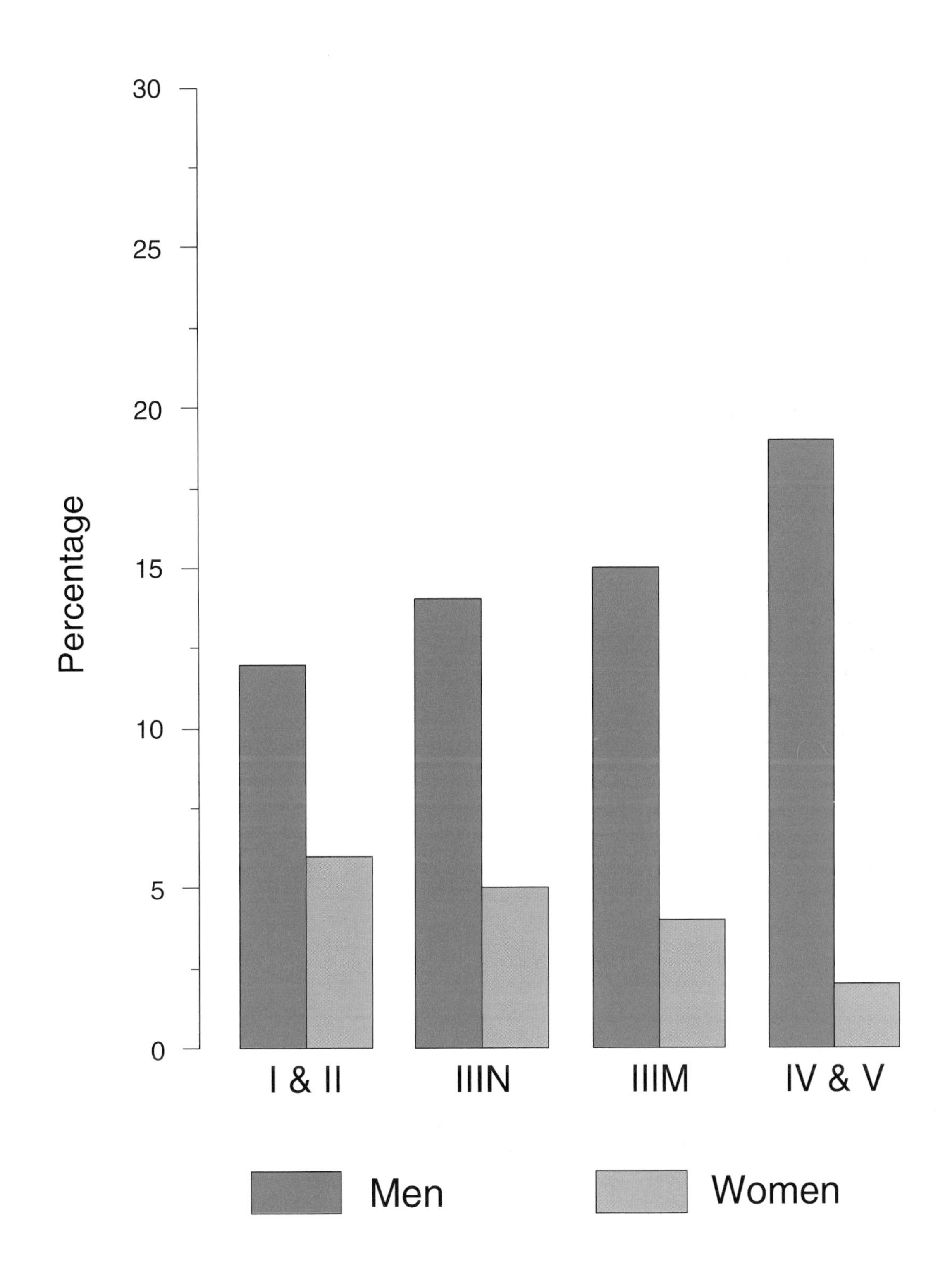

* Social class of head of household
† Regular Participation: 20 minutes at least 3 times a week
Source: HEA/Sports Council,
Allied Dunbar National Fitness Survey

Figure PA4: Participation in Physical Activity of at least moderate intensity
by Social Class, Age 16–74 England 1990/91*

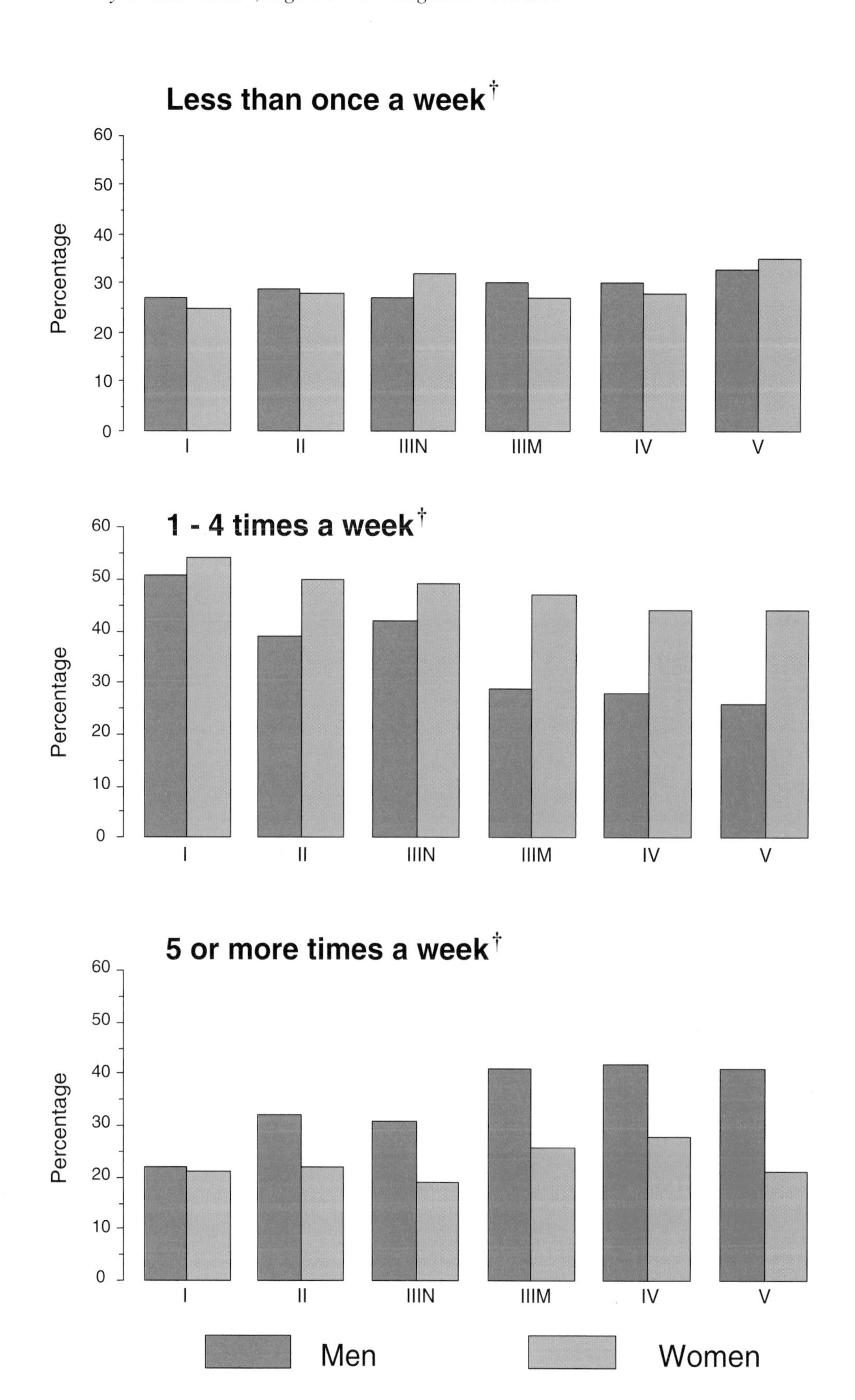

* Social class of head of household
† 30 minutes per occasion
Source: HEA/Sports Council,
Allied Dunbar National Fitness Survey

Figure PA5: Participation in Physical Activity of at least moderate intensity
by Employment Status, Age 16–74 England 1990/91

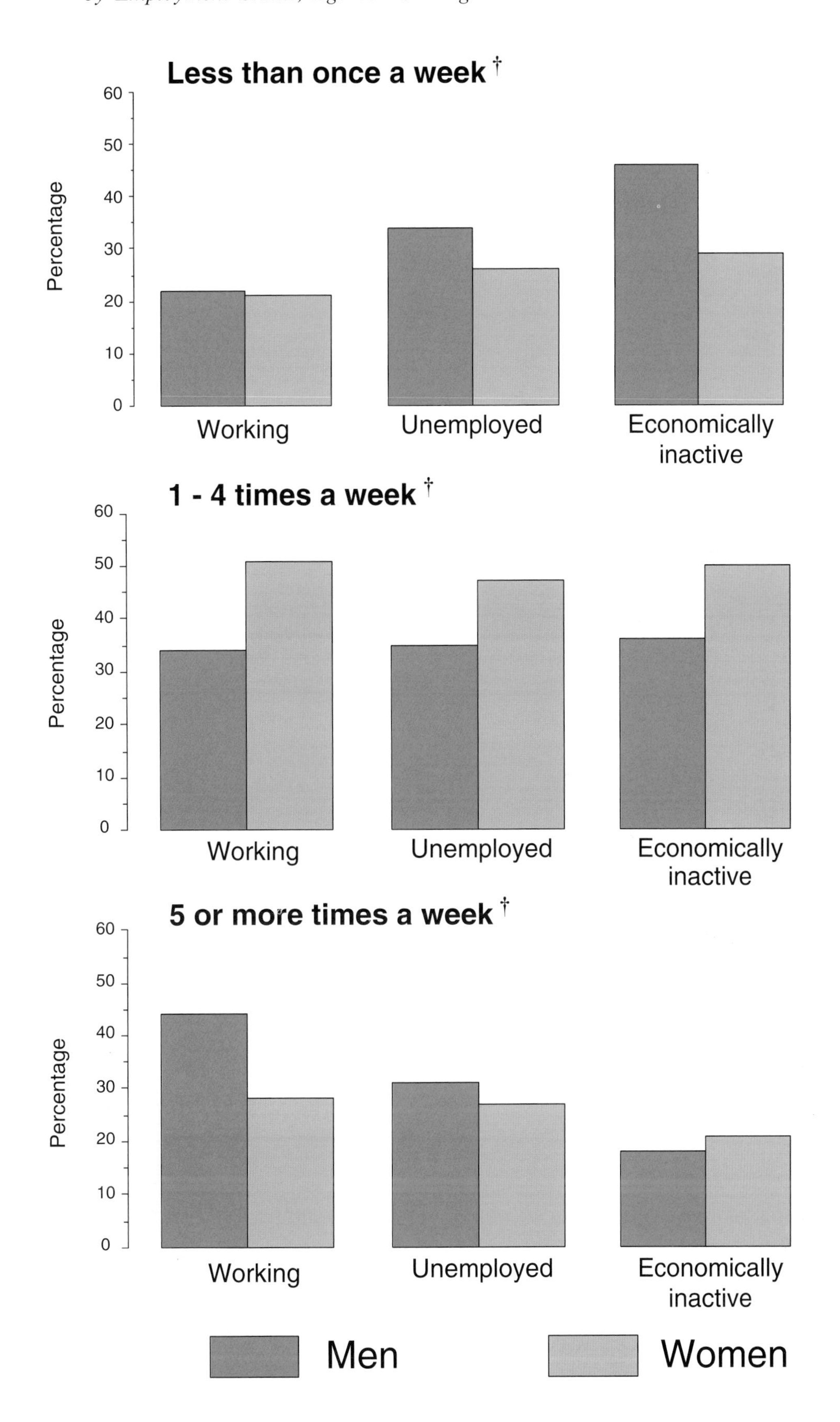

† 30 minutes per occasion
Source: OPCS Health Survey for England

Figure PA6: Regular Participation† in Vigorous Physical Activity
by RHA, Age 16+ England 1993

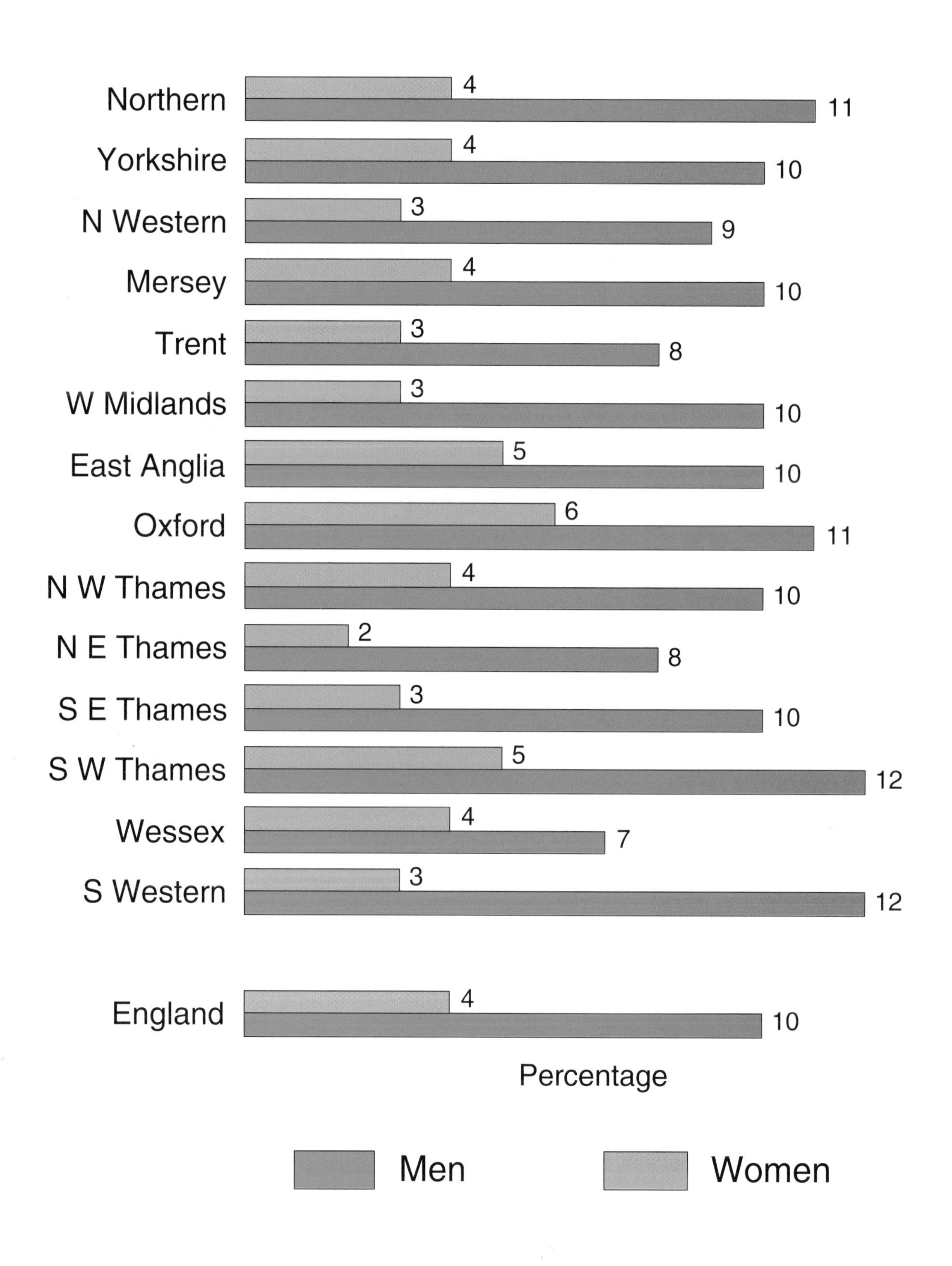

† Regular Participation: 20 minutes at least 3 times a week
Source: OPCS Health Survey for England

CIGARETTE SMOKING

HON Targets:

to reduce the prevalence of cigarette smoking in men and women aged 16 and over to no more than 20% by the year 2000 (a reduction of at least 35% in men and 29% in women, from a prevalence in 1990 of 31% and 28% respectively)

in addition to the overall reduction in prevalence, at least a third of women smokers to stop smoking at the start of their pregnancy by the year 2000

to reduce the consumption of cigarettes by at least 40% by the year 2000 (from 98 billion manufactured cigarettes per year in 1990 to 59 billion)

to reduce smoking prevalence among 11–15 year olds by at least 33% by 1994 (from about 8% in 1988 to less than 6%)

Despite the substantial fall in smoking prevalence over the last twenty years, smoking remains the largest single cause of preventable mortality in England (The Health of the Nation).

The targets for smoking refer to specific behaviour. The baseline percentages come from the General Household Survey and the OPCS surveys of infant feeding and smoking among secondary school children.

Secular trends and variation with age and sex In 1992, 29% of men and 27% of women were cigarette smokers compared with 31% of men and 28% of women in 1990 thus continuing the decline in the prevalence of smoking. In line with this, cigarette consumption has declined since 1989/90 and is projected to continue to decline further. *Figures SM1–2*

People aged 20–24 were the most likely to be smokers (38%). Prevalence then decreased with age to 19% of those aged 60 or more.

The decline in prevalence over time was not standard across all age groups. Among young men (16–24) there has been no decrease since 1988. This is also true of the prevalence of regular smoking among secondary school girls which was the same level in 1993 as in 1982: 11%. There was an overall decrease in smoking among boys from 11% to 8%. *Figures SM3–4*

Socio-economic variation Men and women in the manual socio-economic groups were more likely to be smokers than those in the non-manual groups. Differential rates of decline in the prevalence of smoking between these groups resulted in the differences becoming larger, so that in 1992 the prevalence among men in the unskilled manual group was three times as high as among those in the professional group (41% compared with 13%). The difference for women was slightly smaller. *Figure SM5*

An HEA survey of smoking among 9 to 15 year olds found no social class differences in that age group.

There was a strong social class gradient in the proportions of women smokers who stopped smoking during pregnancy. Overall, in 1990, 27% of women who smoked before pregnancy, stopped during pregnancy. The proportions varied from 50% and 41% of those in groups I and II to 24% and 17% of those in groups IV and V, among whom pre-pregnancy smoking was already much more prevalent. These variations serve to amplify the social class gradient in the prevalence of smoking among pregnant women. Among pregnant women in social class V the prevalence of smoking was five times as high as among pregnant women in social class I (39% and 8%). *Figure SM6*

Employment status One in two unemployed men (51%) were smokers compared with 29% of men who were working. The difference for women was smaller. *Figure SM7*

Marital status Married men and women were less likely to smoke than their unmarried counterparts with the highest prevalence (36%) found among men who were widowed, divorced or separated. *Figure SM8*

Ethnic group Prevalence of smoking also showed considerable variation between ethnic groups. In 1992, an HEA survey of ethnic minority groups found that 40% of Bangladeshi men were smokers compared with 19% of Indian men and 28% of both Pakistani and African Caribbean men. Very few Asian women were smokers. *Figure SM9*

Among 9 to 15 year olds, 6% of white children were regular smokers compared with 2% of both Asian and African-Caribbean children.

Geographical variation In comparison with these personal socio-demographic indicators the variation in smoking prevalence with geographical area was small. Within England, smoking prevalence varied with respect to region but, among men, showed no general trend across the country. Among women the prevalence of smoking was generally higher in the northern regions. *Figure SM10*

There was little variation with region in the prevalence of smoking among secondary school children; in 1993, 9% of 11 to 15 year olds in the north were regular smokers compared with 11% in the Midlands, 9% in the South and 8% in Greater London.

The prevalence of smoking in both Wales and Scotland was higher than in England for men and women. Among secondary school children, however, there was little variation for the boys but regular smoking was more prevalent among Scottish girls (13% compared with 10% in England and 9% in Wales). *Table SM1*

References and Notes

OPCS. General Household Survey 1992, London HMSO 1994 (Series GHS; no. 23) GB. Age 16+

OPCS. Smoking among Secondary School Children in England 1993, London HMSO 1994 Age 11–15

OPCS. Smoking among Secondary School Children in 1992, London HMSO 1993 Contains data for Scotland and Wales Age 11–15

DH Statistical Bulletin 1994/14. Statistics on smoking England 1974 to 1993 Reanalysis of GHS data for England

OPCS Infant Feeding 1990 London HMSO 1992

HEA. Black and Minority Ethnic Groups in England, HEA 1994 Age 16–74

HEA. Tomorrow's Young Adults, HEA 1992 England 1989 Age 9–15

Figure SM1A: Cigarette Smokers in the Population
by Sex, All Ages England 1974–1992

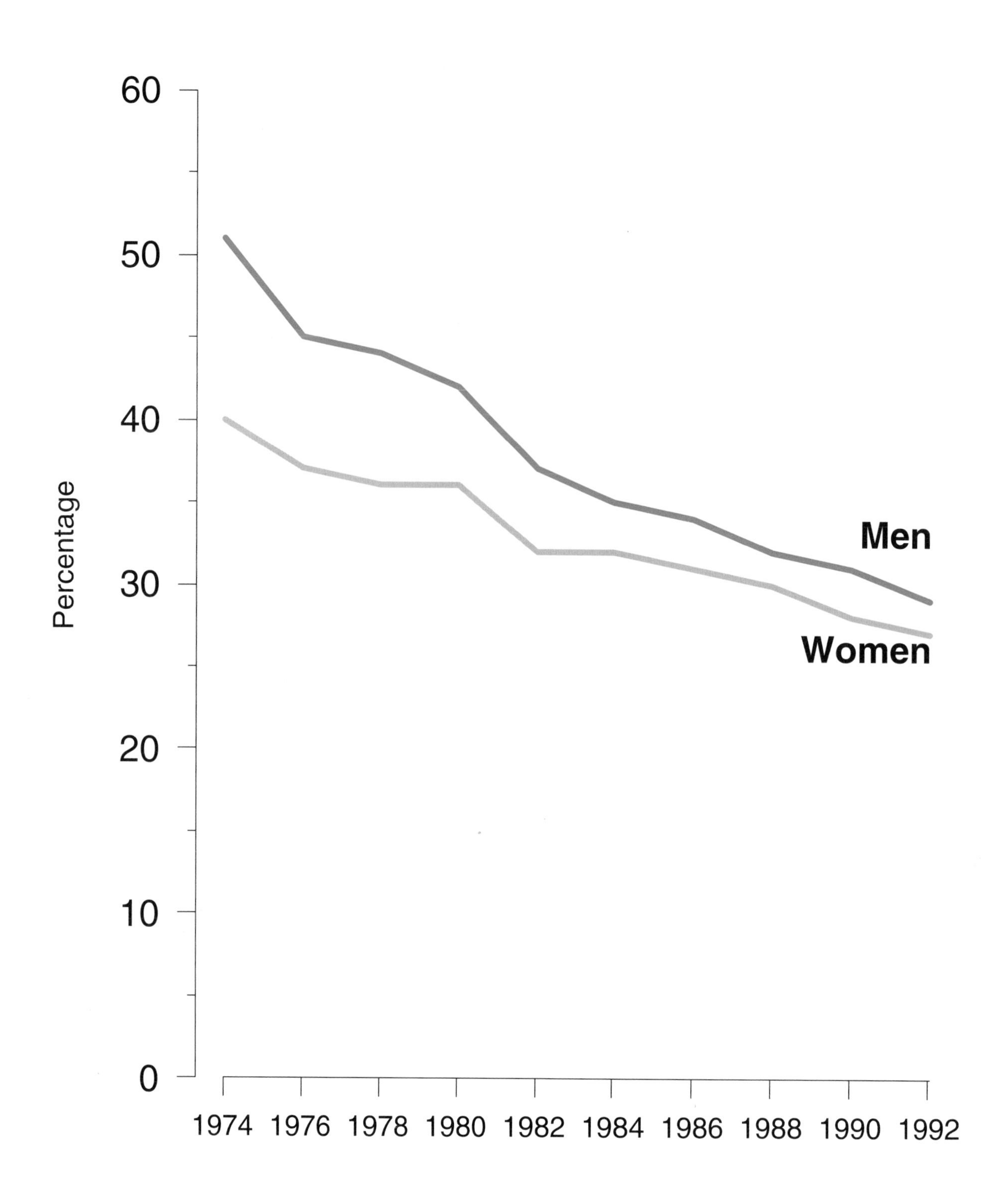

Source: OPCS General Household Survey

Figure SM1B: Cigarette Smokers in the Population
by Sex and Age England 1974–1992

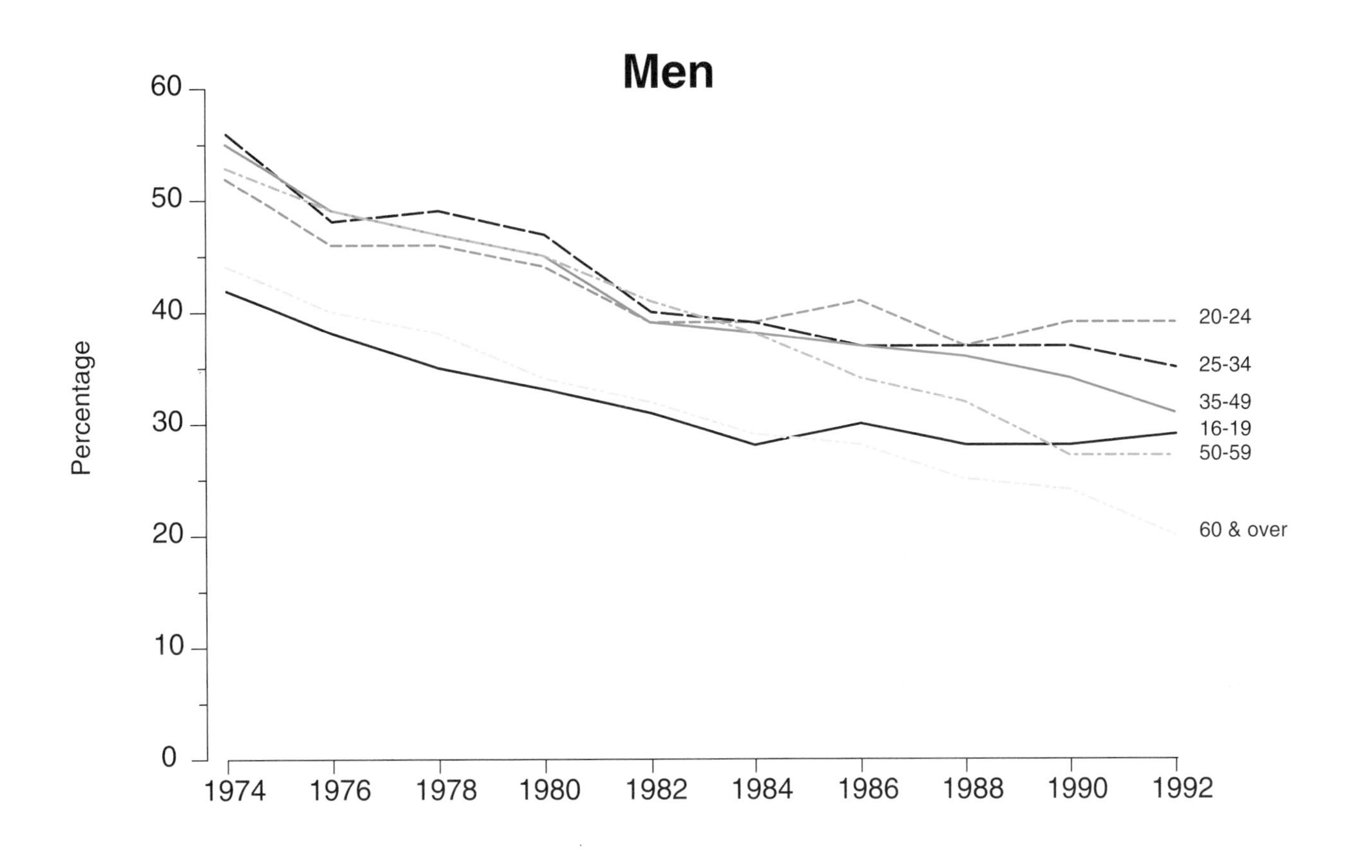

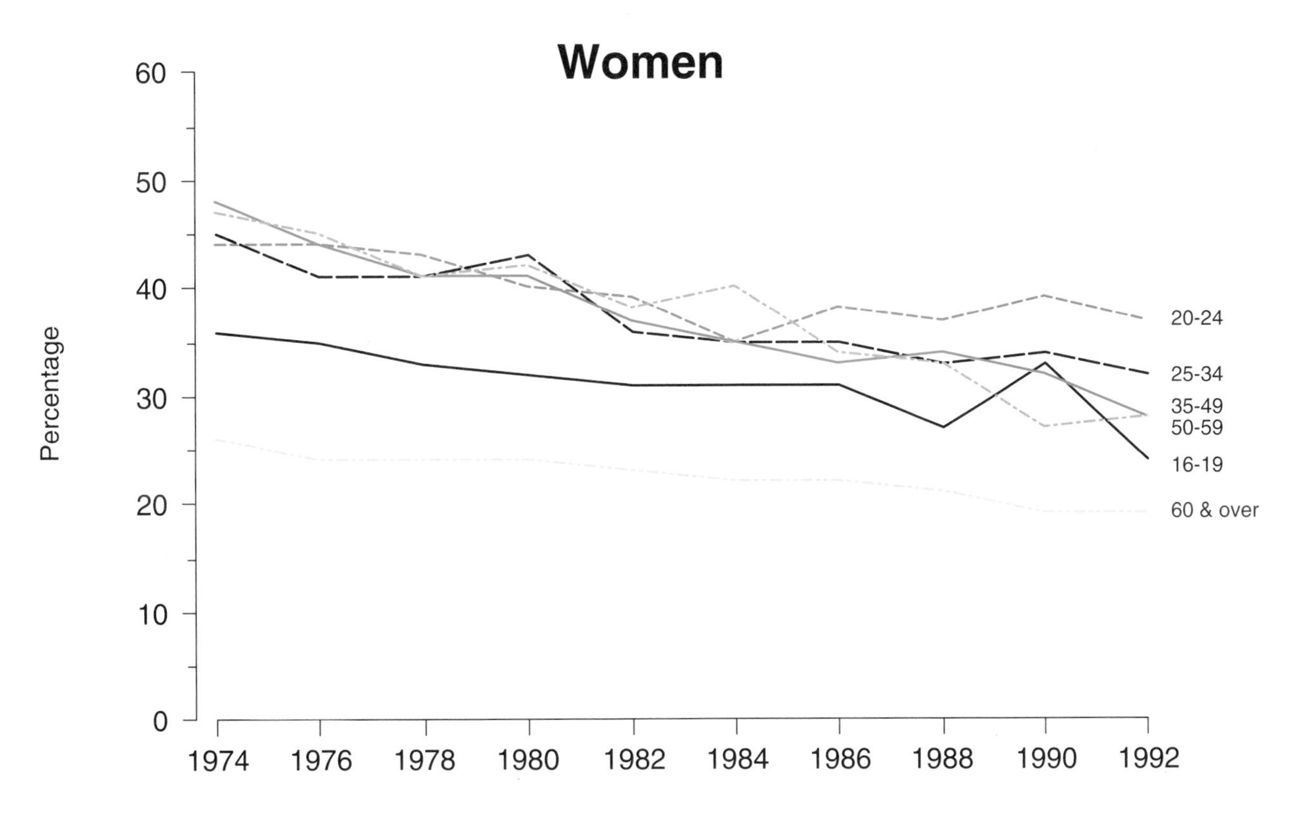

Source: OPCS General Household Survey

Figure SM2: Cigarette Released for Home Consumption
United Kingdom 1981/82–1993/94 and target for year 2000

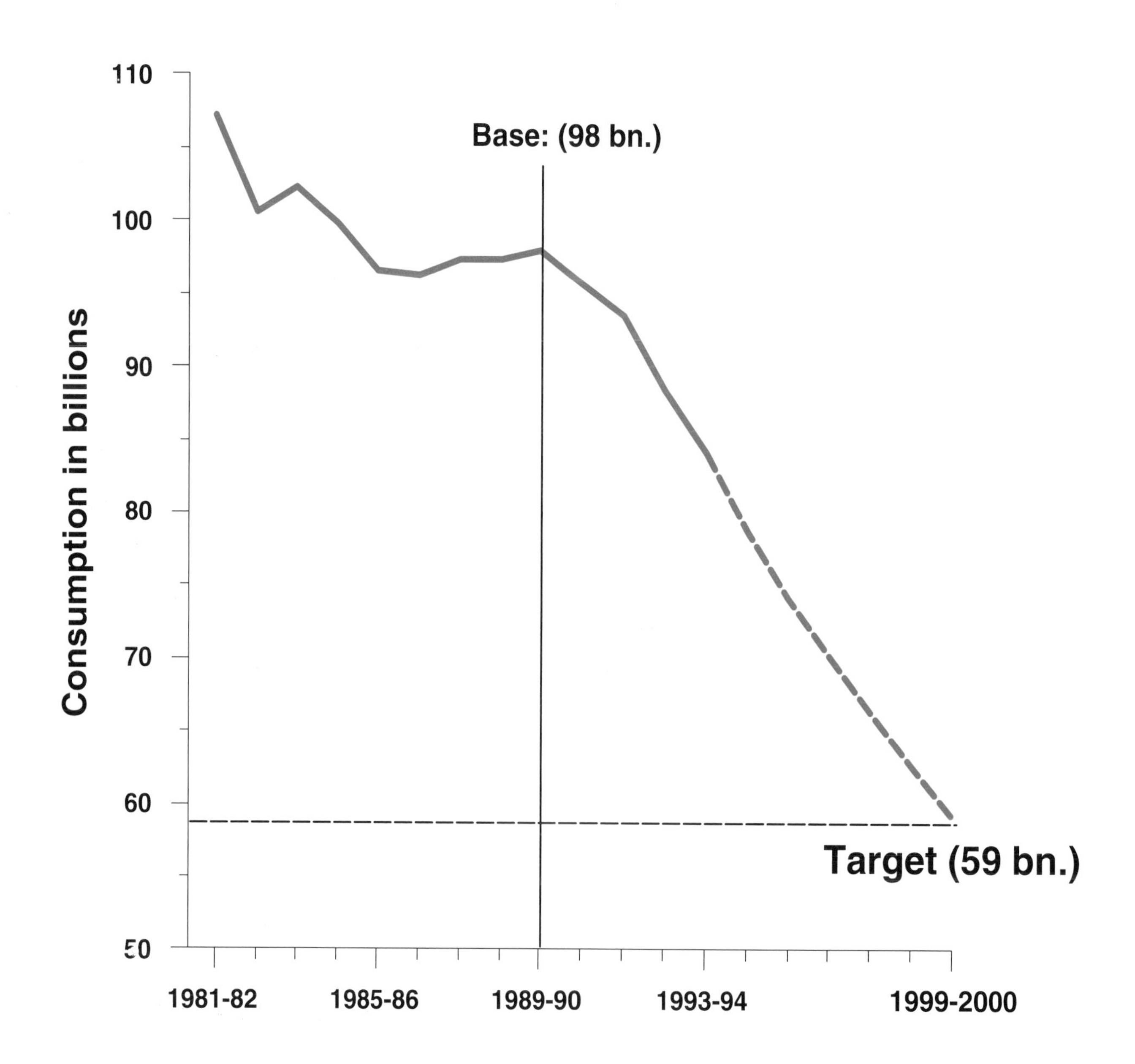

Source: HM Customs & Excise

Figure SM3: Smoking Among Secondary School Children
by Age England 1982–1993

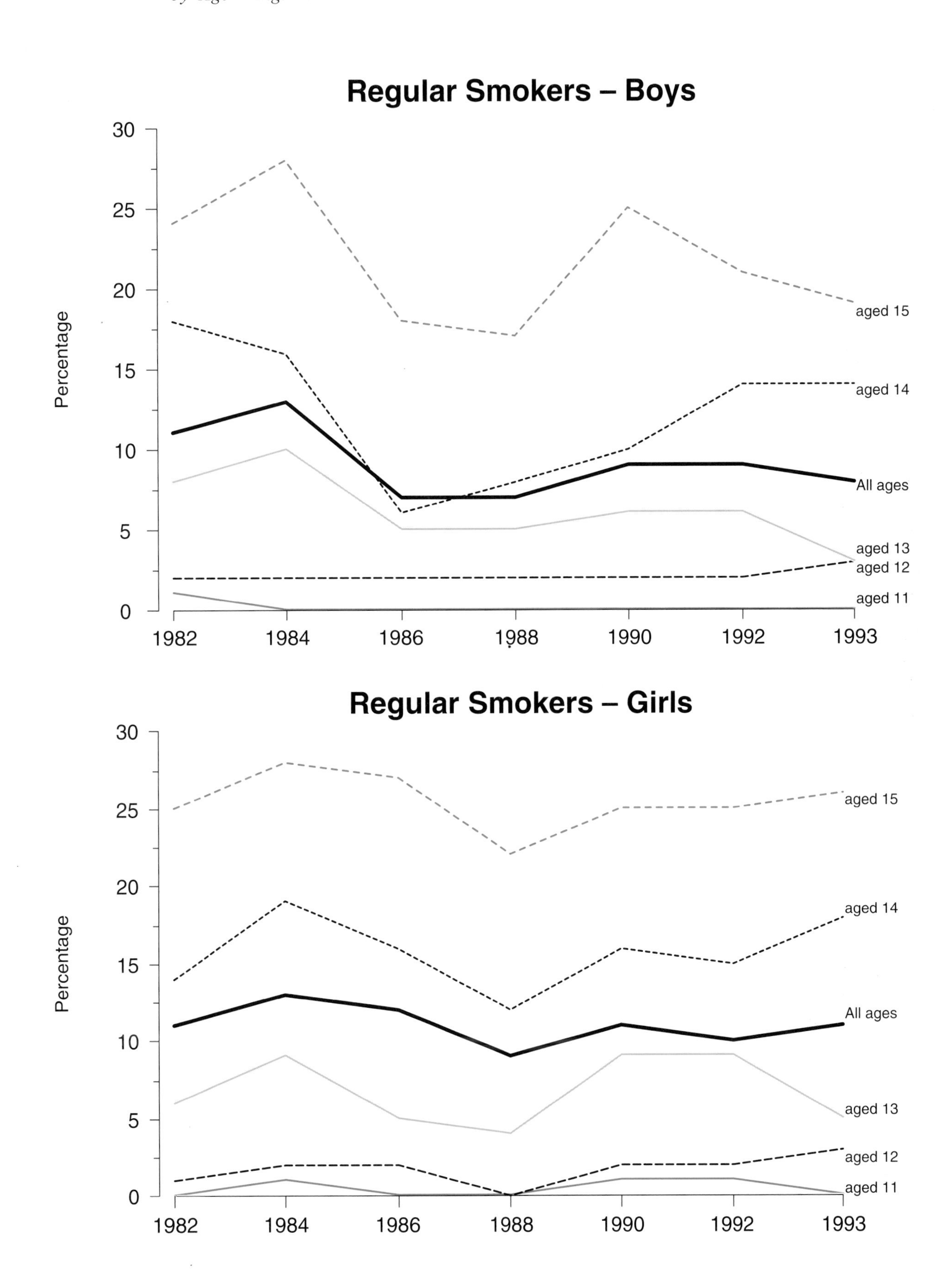

Regular smokers defined as smoking 1 or more cigarettes per week

Source: OPCS Smoking among Secondary School Children in 1993

Figure SM4: Smoking Among Secondary School Children
by Age England 1993

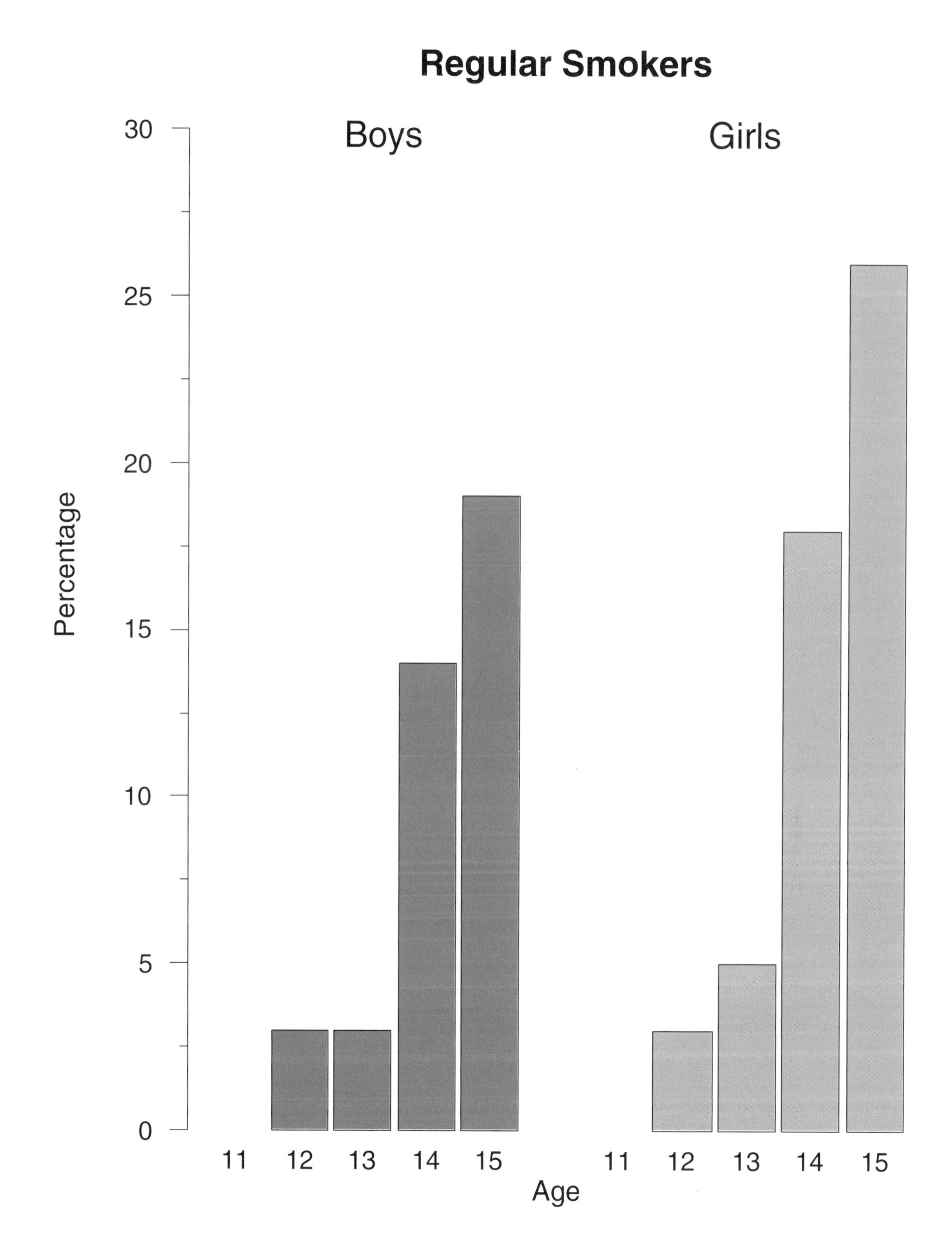

Regular smokers defined as smoking 1 or more cigarettes per week
Source: OPCS Smoking among Secondary School Children in 1993

Figure SM5: Prevalence of Cigarette Smokers
by SEG, Age 16+ Great Britain 1974 England 1990 and 1992

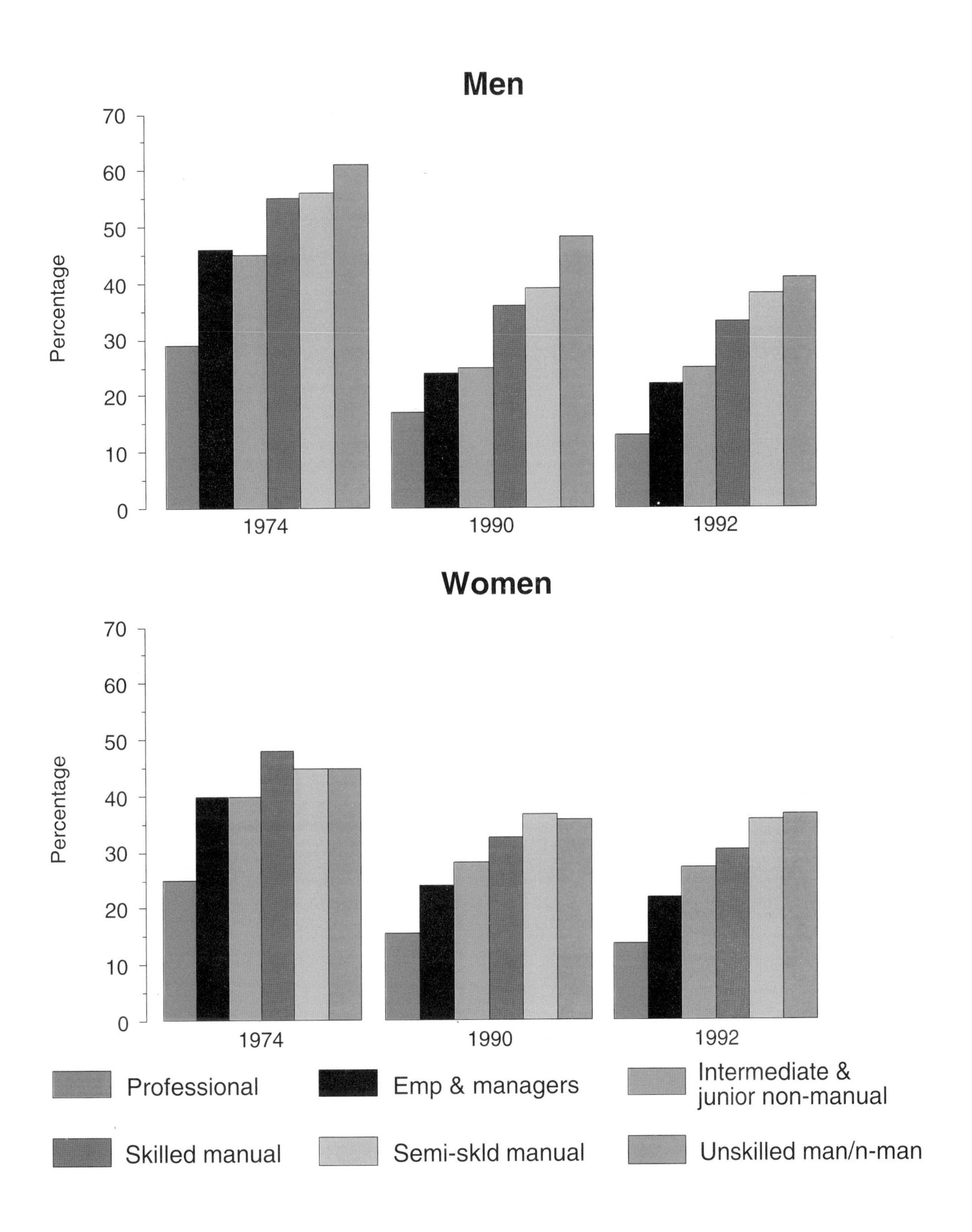

Source: General Household Survey, analysis by Statistics Division 2D

Figure SM6: Mothers Smoking before & during Pregnancy
by Social Class, Age 16+ Great Britain 1985 & 1990

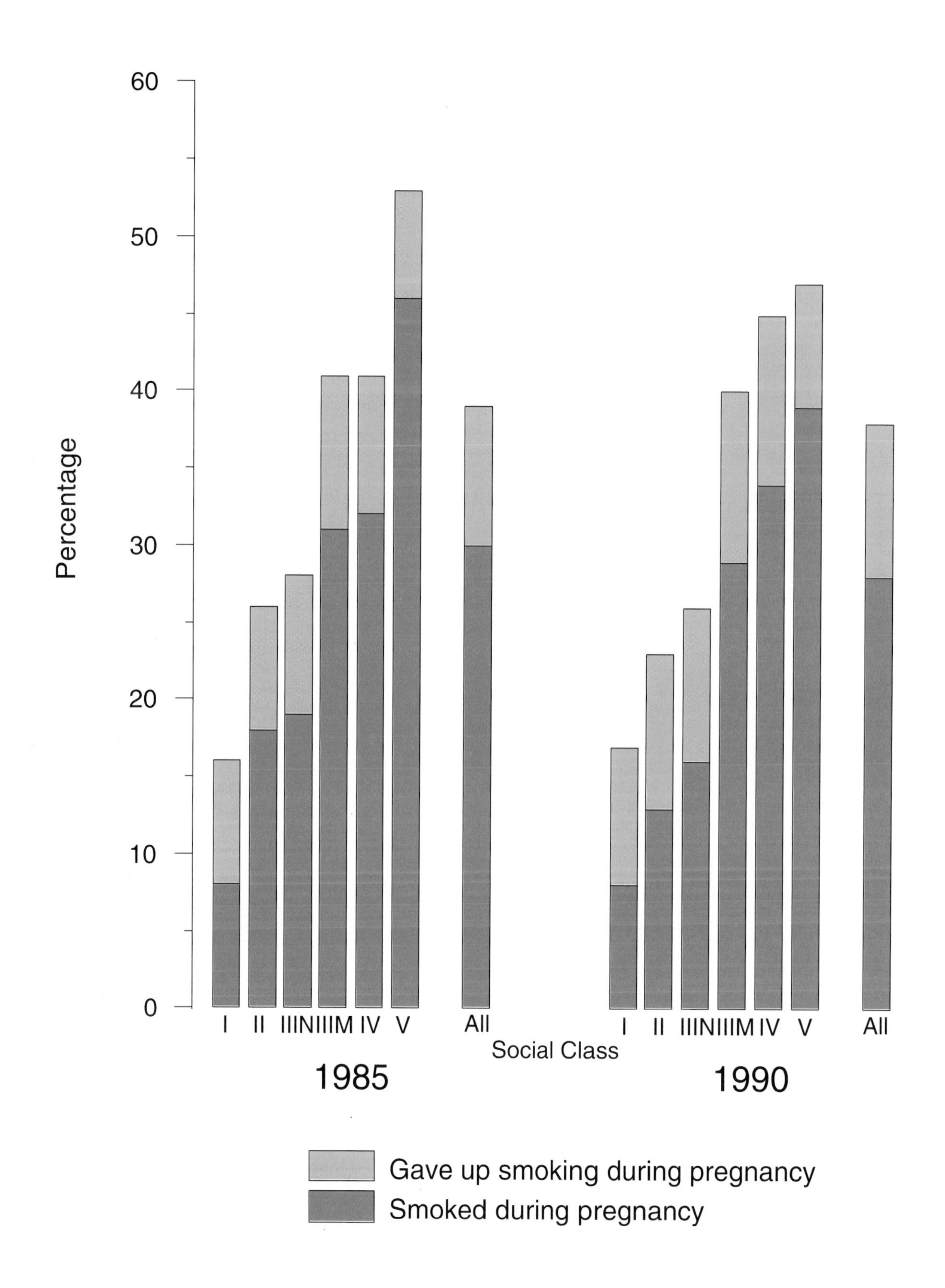

Source: OPCS Smoking Infant Feeding 1990

Figure SM7: Prevalence of Cigarette Smokers
by Economic Status, Age 16–59 Great Britain 1992

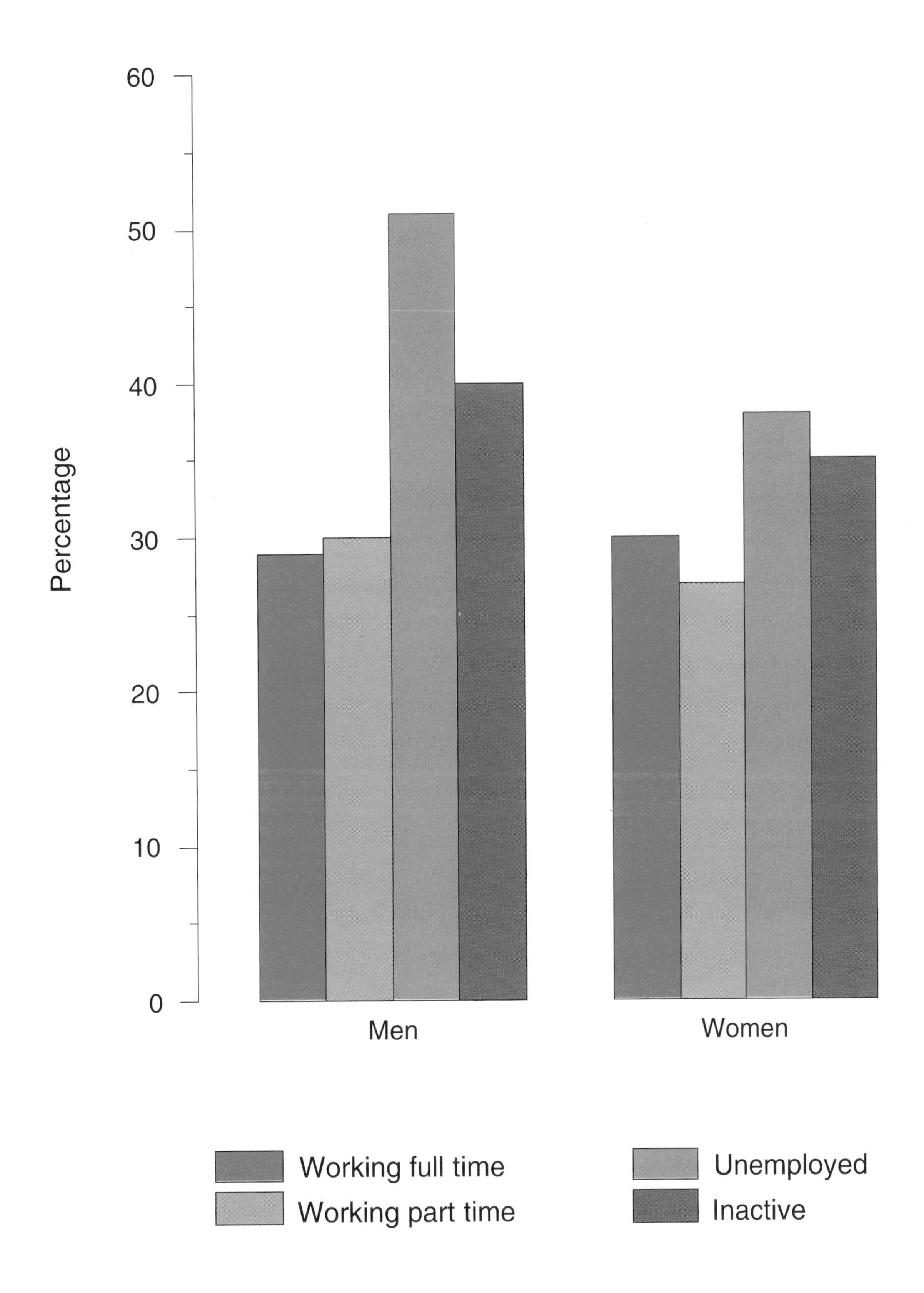

Source: OPCS General Household Survey

Figure SM8: Prevalence of Cigarette Smokers
by Marital Status, Age 16+ Great Britain 1992

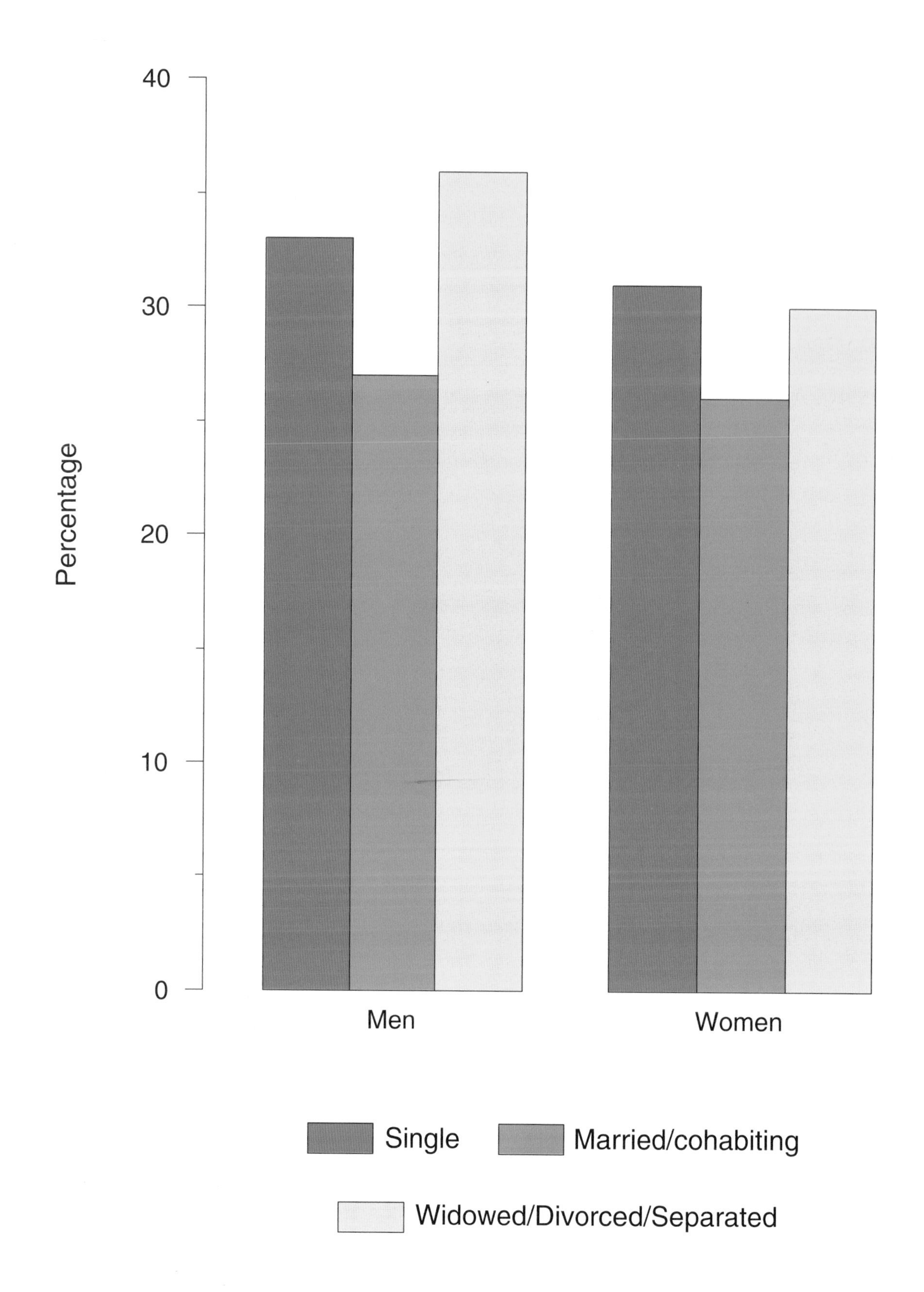

Source: OPCS General Household Survey

Figure SM9: Prevalence of Cigarette Smokers
by Ethnicity, Age 16+ England 1992

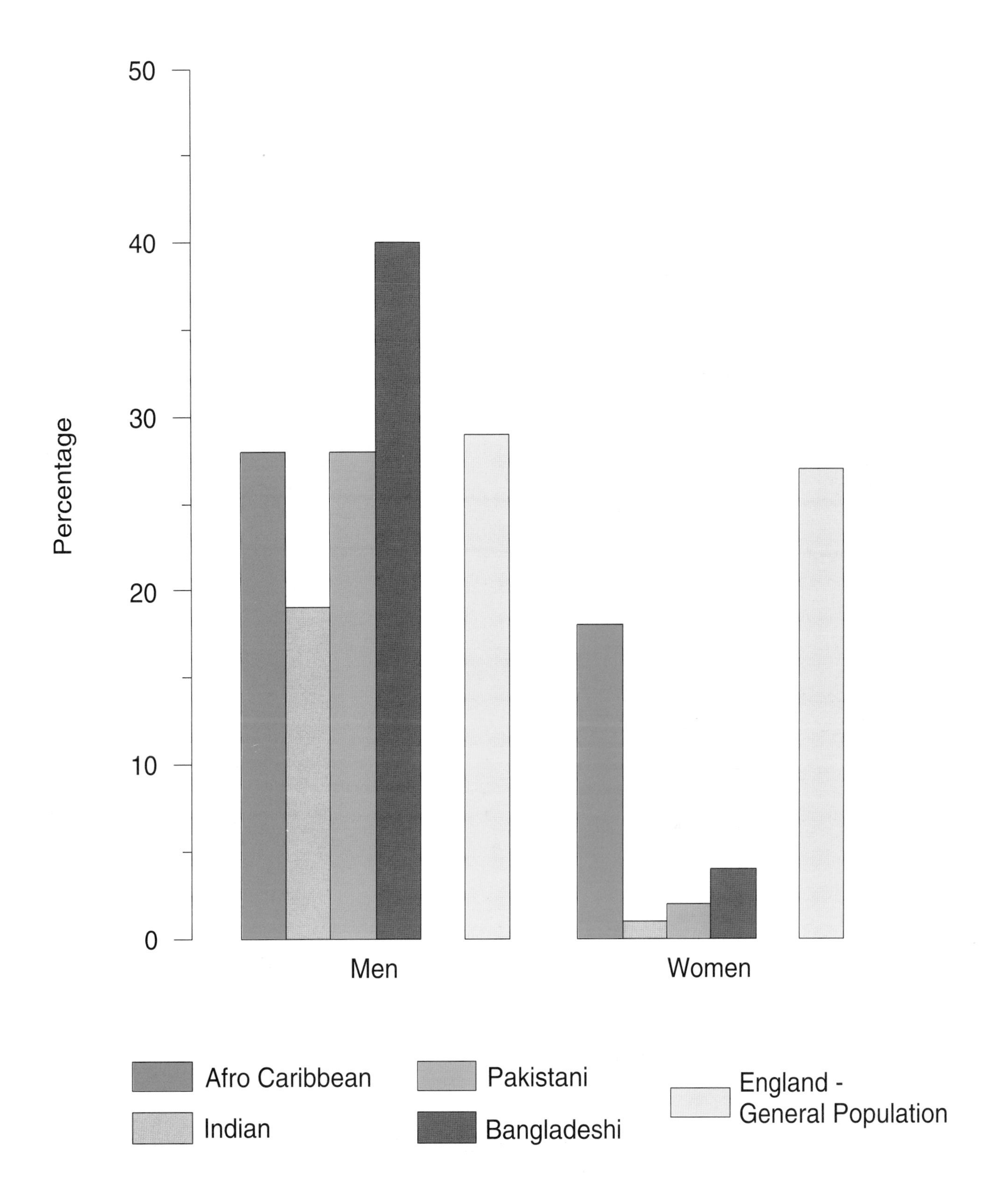

Source: HEA Black & Minority Ethnic Groups in England
OPCS General Household Survey

Figure SM10: Prevalence of Cigarette Smokers
by RHA, Age 16+ England 1992

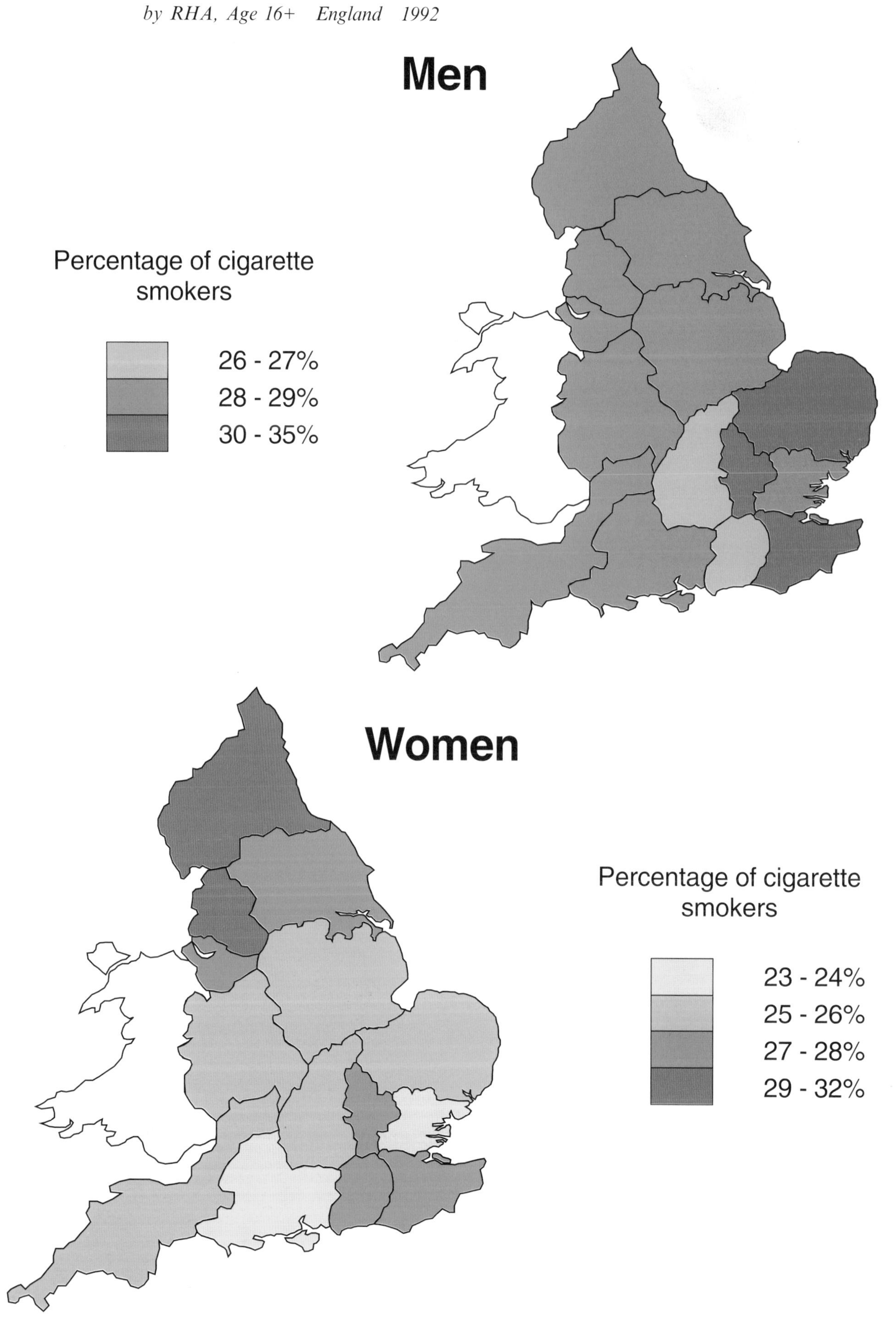

Source: OPCS General Household Survey

Table SM1 *Prevalence of smoking in England, Scotland and Wales 1992*

	England	Scotland	Wales	Great Britain
Prevalence of smoking				
Men	29% *7,284*	34% *721*	32% *412*	29% *8,417*
Women	27% *8,379*	34% *886*	33% *499*	28% *9,764*
Regular smokers				
Boys	9% *1,662*	10% *1,489*	9% *1,394*	*
Girls	10% *1,626*	13% *1,411*	9% *1,385*	*

Source: OPCS GHS and Smoking among secondary school children

SCREENING FOR CANCER

HON Targets:

> to reduce the death rate for breast cancer in the population invited for screening by at least 25% by the year 2000 (from 95.1 per 100,000 population in 1990 to no more than 71.3 per 100,000)
>
> to reduce the incidence of invasive cervical cancer by at least 20% by the year 2000 (from 15 per 100,000 population in 1986 to no more than 12 per 100,000)

The national breast cancer screening programme invites women aged 50–64 to be screened every three years. Attendance for screening when invited, among women aged 50–64, is the behavioural indicator used in this overview. The data comes from the Korner return KC62.

In the national cervical cancer screening programme health authorities are required to invite women aged 20–64 for cervical screening and to recall them at least every five years. Information is obtained from the Korner return KC53 and there are data relating to the coverage of women aged 20–64 in the past 5½ years and also the response to invitations to screening each year. The response to invitation is used as the behavioural indicator in this overview.

Risk factors for cervical cancer include age at first intercourse, number of partners and condom use. These behaviours are included within the key area of sexual health.

Secular trends and variation with age Among women aged 50–64, 72% responded to an invitation to breast screening in 1992/93, the same as in 1991/92.

In 1992/93, 64% of women aged 20–64 invited to cervical screening were screened. Response to the invitation was highest among women aged 35–39 (72%) and lowest among those aged 20–24 (49%). *Figure SC1*

Data on trends in *uptake* of cervical screening invitations each year were not available but the figures for coverage of the target age group (20–64) in the past 5½ years show an increase from 43% in 1988/89 to 83% in 1992/93. (See notes below for definitions.)

Geographical variation The common feature of the regional variation in uptake of invitations to either breast or cervical screening was the lower response in the Thames regions. It is suggested that this may be more a reflection of problems with calling women to screening rather than the women's response. Women in East Anglia and Trent were the most likely to take up an invitation to breast screening while those in Yorkshire and Mersey were considerably more likely than women elsewhere to attend for cervical screening. *Figures SC2–3*

Ethnic group In 1992, the HEA survey of ethnic minority groups asked women aged 16–74 if they had ever had a cervical smear test and if so how long ago it was. In the comparative UK sample 77% said they had been screened in the past five years which corresponds well with the official figure of 83%. Screening among African-Caribbean women was similar to the UK survey figure (81%) but the figures for the South Asian women are considerably lower: 63% of Indian women reported having a smear test in the past five years, 45% of Pakistani women and only 33% of Bangladeshi women. *Table SC1*

The same survey also asked indirectly about screening for breast cancer. Although the researchers on the survey suggest that the figures are underestimates, they indicate that the take up of breast screening is lower among Asian women, and in particular Bangladeshi women, than for the general population.

References and Notes

Breast and cervical. The percentage response to invitations to screening each year is based on the number of women invited to screening.

Cervical. The percentage coverage in the past five years is based on the number of women aged 20–64 resident less those women who have ceased to be recalled.

Both of the following reports are produced by DH Statistics Division 2B DH. Breast Cancer Screening 1992–93 Summary Information from Form KC62 England DH. Cervical Cytology 1992–93 Summary Information from Form KC53 England

HEA. Black and Minority Ethnic Groups in England, HEA 1994. This report also gives UK figures from the HEA Health and Lifestyle Survey 1992

Figure SC1: Cervical Screening Uptake of Invitation
by Age England 1992/93

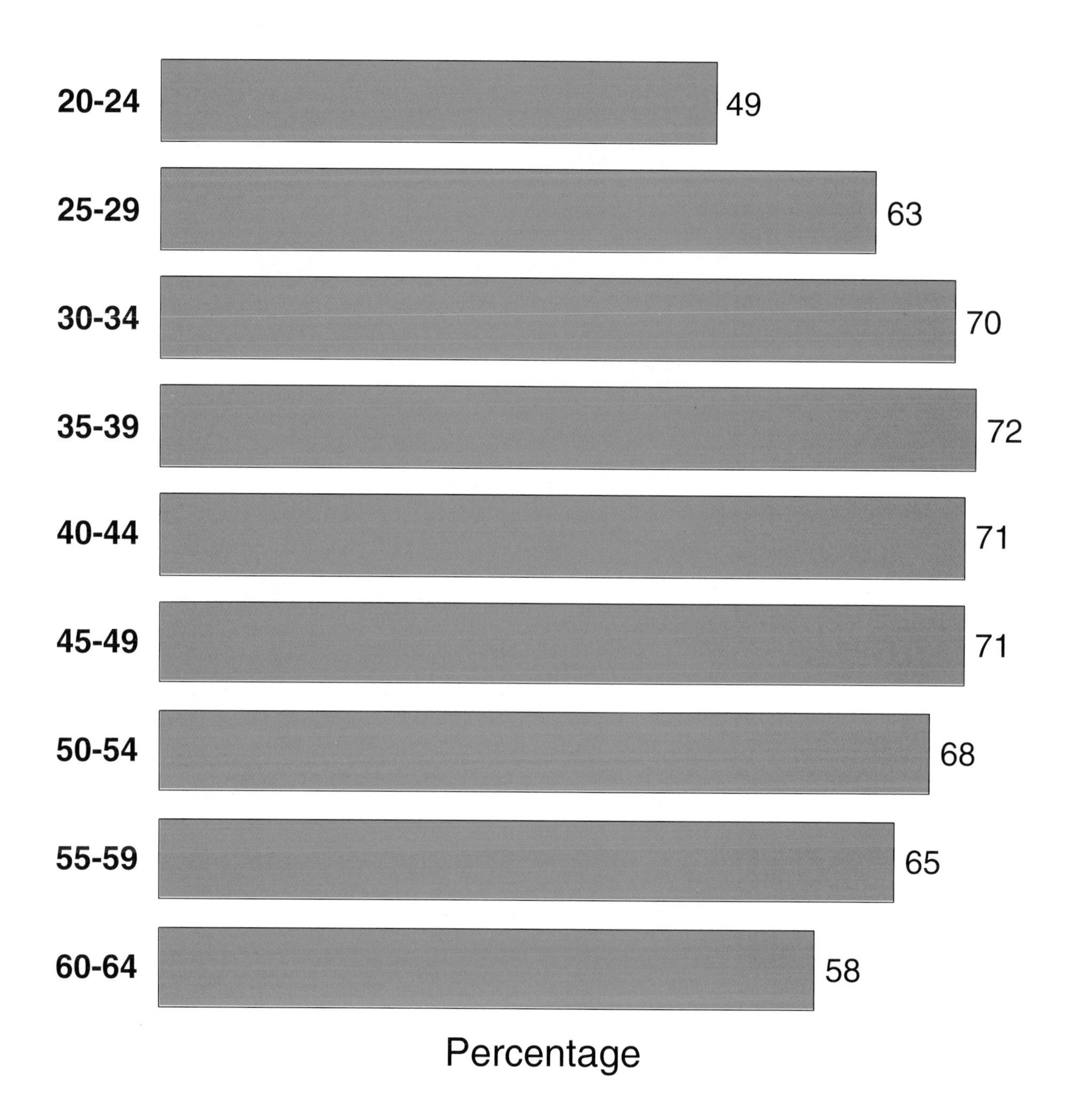

Source: DH Summary Information from Form KC53

Figure SC2: Breast Screening, Uptake of Invitation
by RHA, Age 50–64 England 1992/93

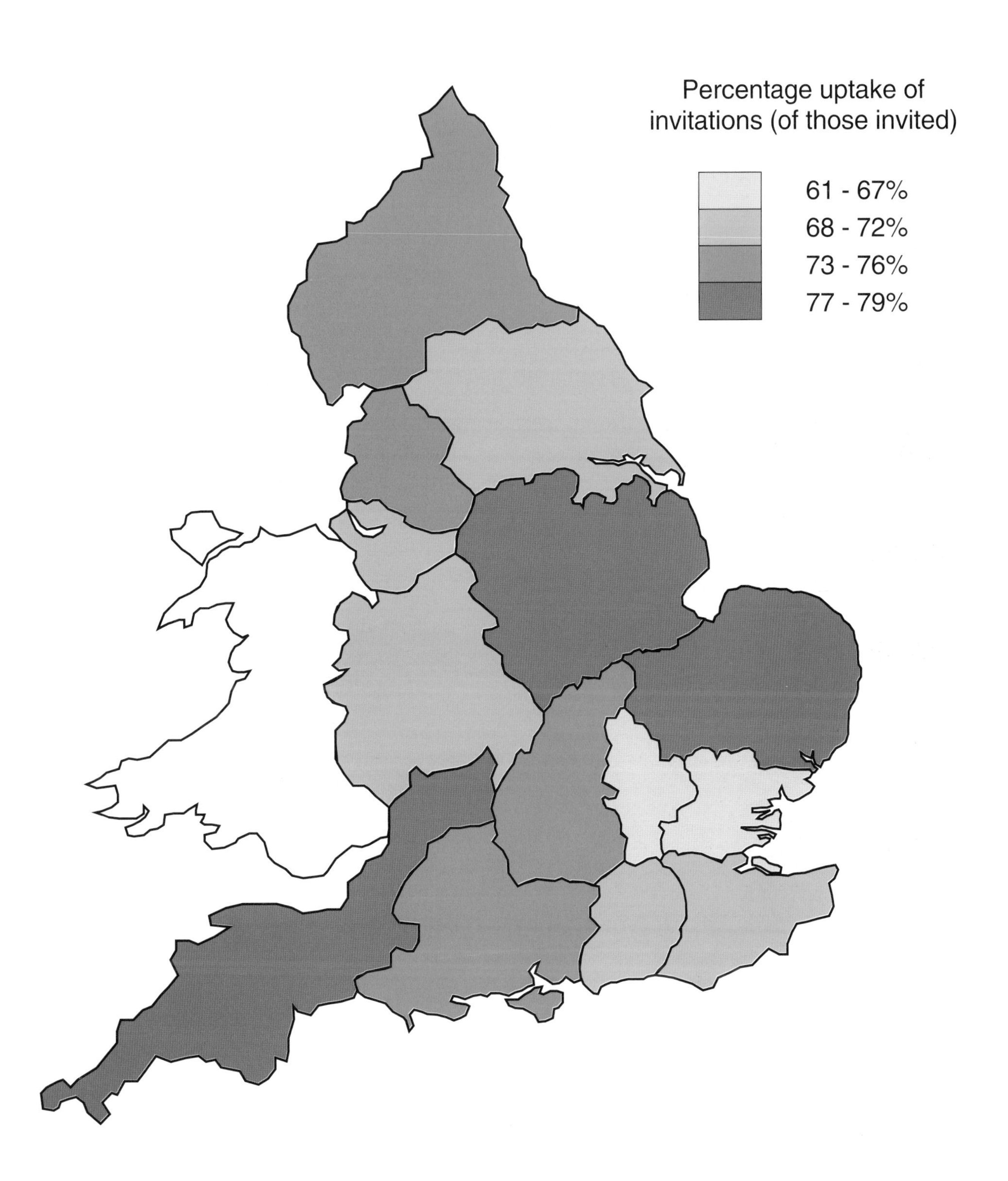

Source: DH Summary Information from Form KC62

Figure SC3: Cervical Screening, Uptake of Invitation
by RHA, Age 20–64 England 1992/93

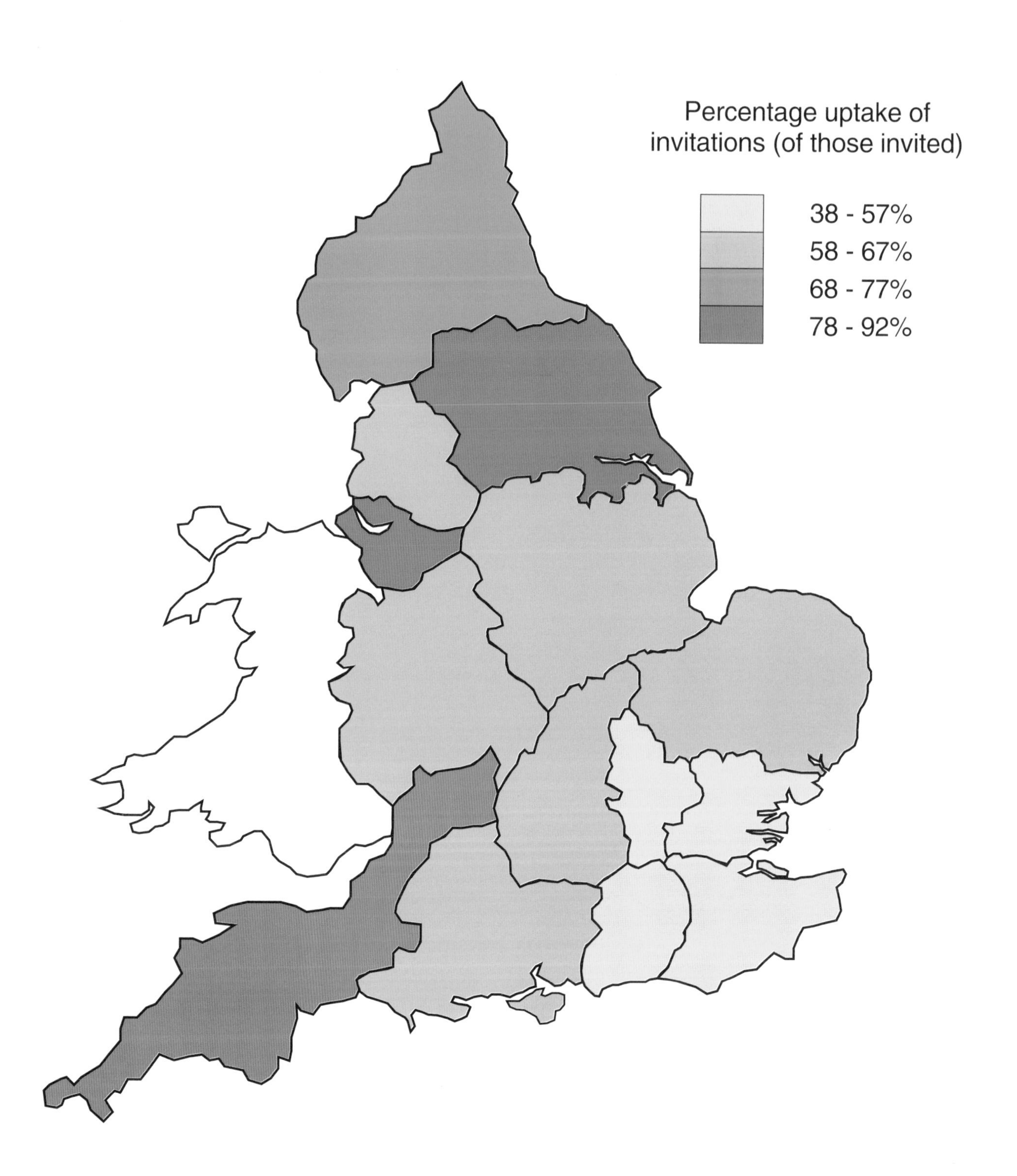

Source: DH Summary Information from Form KC53

Table SC1 *Proportion of women aged 16–74 who reported having a cervical smear test in the past five years*

UK General Population	African-Carribbean	Indian	Pakistani	Bangladeshi
77%	81%	63%	45%	33%

Source: HEA Black and Minority Ethnic Groups in England

EXCESSIVE SUN EXPOSURE

> HON Target:
>
> to halt the year-on-year increase in the incidence of skin cancer by 2005

The HON cites exposure to the sun as the main risk factor for skin cancer; prevalence of sunburn is used as an indicator of risk. Although not an actual behaviour, it can also be used as an indicator of excessive sun exposure.

The data source is a series of questions asked on the OPCS Omnibus Survey (see notes).

Secular trends and variation with age and sex In 1993, 39% of men and 34% of women reported at least one episode of sunburn in the past year. For 16% of men and 14% of women the episodes involved more than reddening of the skin which lasted overnight. The proportion reporting any episodes of sunburn decreased with age from 57% of men aged 16–24 to 23% aged 55 and over with equivalent figures for women of 62% and 15%. Older people were also less likely to experience serious sunburn. No trend data are currently available. *Figure SB1*

Socio-economic status Women in social classes I and II were more likely than other women to report sunburn but the differences between the proportions reporting more serious sunburn were smaller. There was no significant social class variation for men. *Figure SB2*

Employment status Sunburn was unrelated to employment status.

Marital status Single men and women were more likely to report at least one episode of sunburn in the past year than married men and women (47% compared with 39% for men and 53% compared with 34% for women). This variation was also found for serious sunburn among women but not for men. *Figure SB3*

Family status The prevalence of sunburn was higher among married people with children than those without – 46% of married women with children reported at least one episode of sunburn in the past year compared with 29% of married women with no children – but the differences in the prevalence of serious sunburn were not so great. Prevalence of sunburn was lowest among people living in single person households which partly reflected the older age profile of this group. *Figure SB4*

Geographical variation Sunburn varied slightly with geographical region among men but there was no north-south trend. There was no significant variation among women.

References and Notes

Data for the prevalence of sunburn come from a series of questions asked in the OPCS Omnibus Survey in October 1993. These questions have been repeated in January 1995

'During the last 12 months how many times have you had the following types of sunburn

A. Sunburn causing reddening of the skin that lasted overnight but with no skin soreness

B. Reddening and soreness of the skin lasting for 1–2 days but no blistering

C. Reddening and soreness of the skin lasting for more than 2 days but no blistering

D. Reddening and soreness of the skin lasting for more than 2 days together with blistering'

Any episodes of the above were included in the definition of sunburn. More serious sunburn included any episodes of B to D. The sample size for this analysis is 1,920 people.

Melia J, Bulman A 'Sunburn and tanning in a British population' Journal of Public Health Medicine 1995 vol 17 pp 223–229

Figure SB1: Prevalence of Sunburn†

by Age & Sex Great Britain 1993

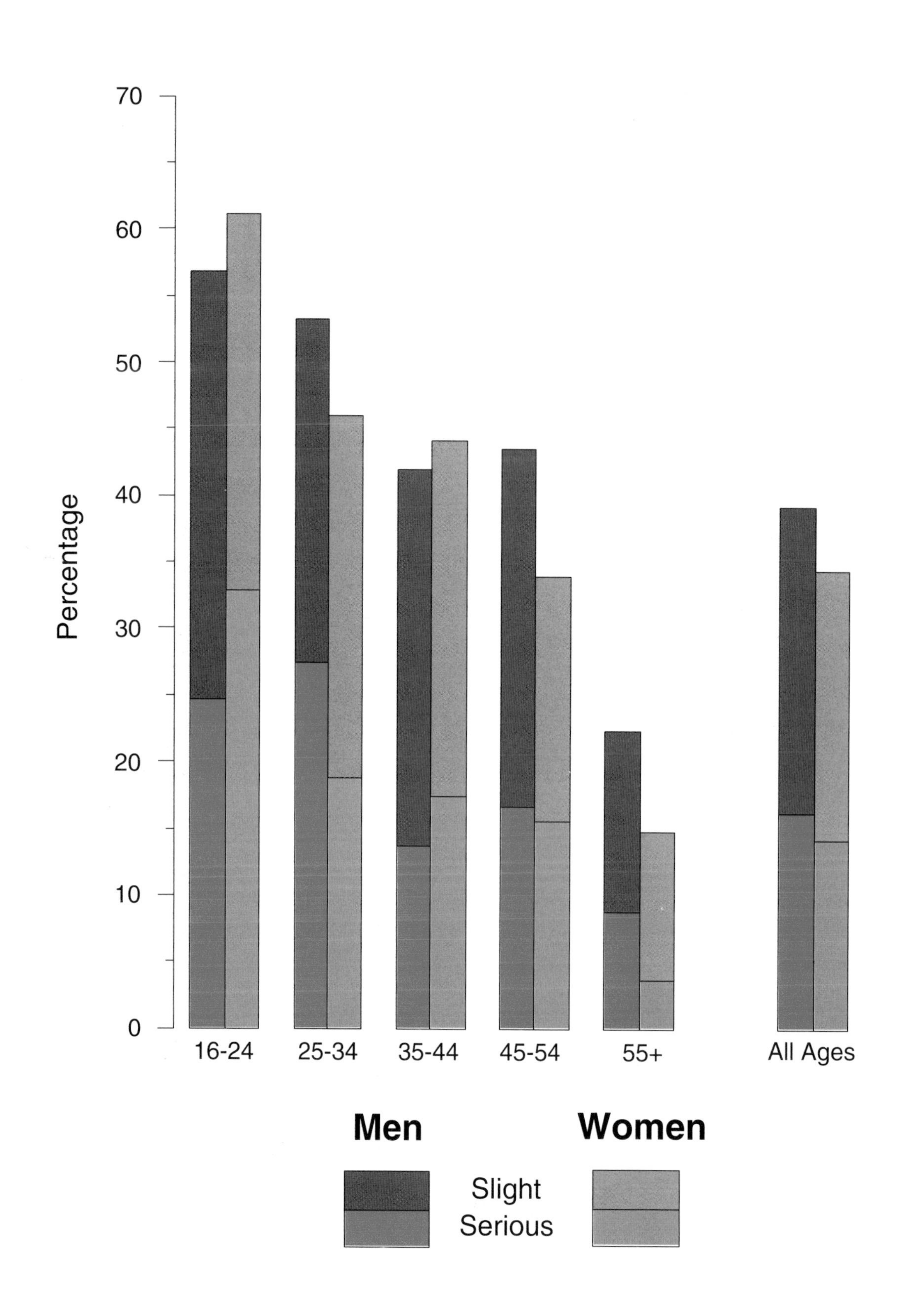

† Experienced in the past 12 months

Source: OPCS Omnibus Survey

Figure SB2: Prevalence of Sunburn†
by Social Class & Sex Great Britain 1993

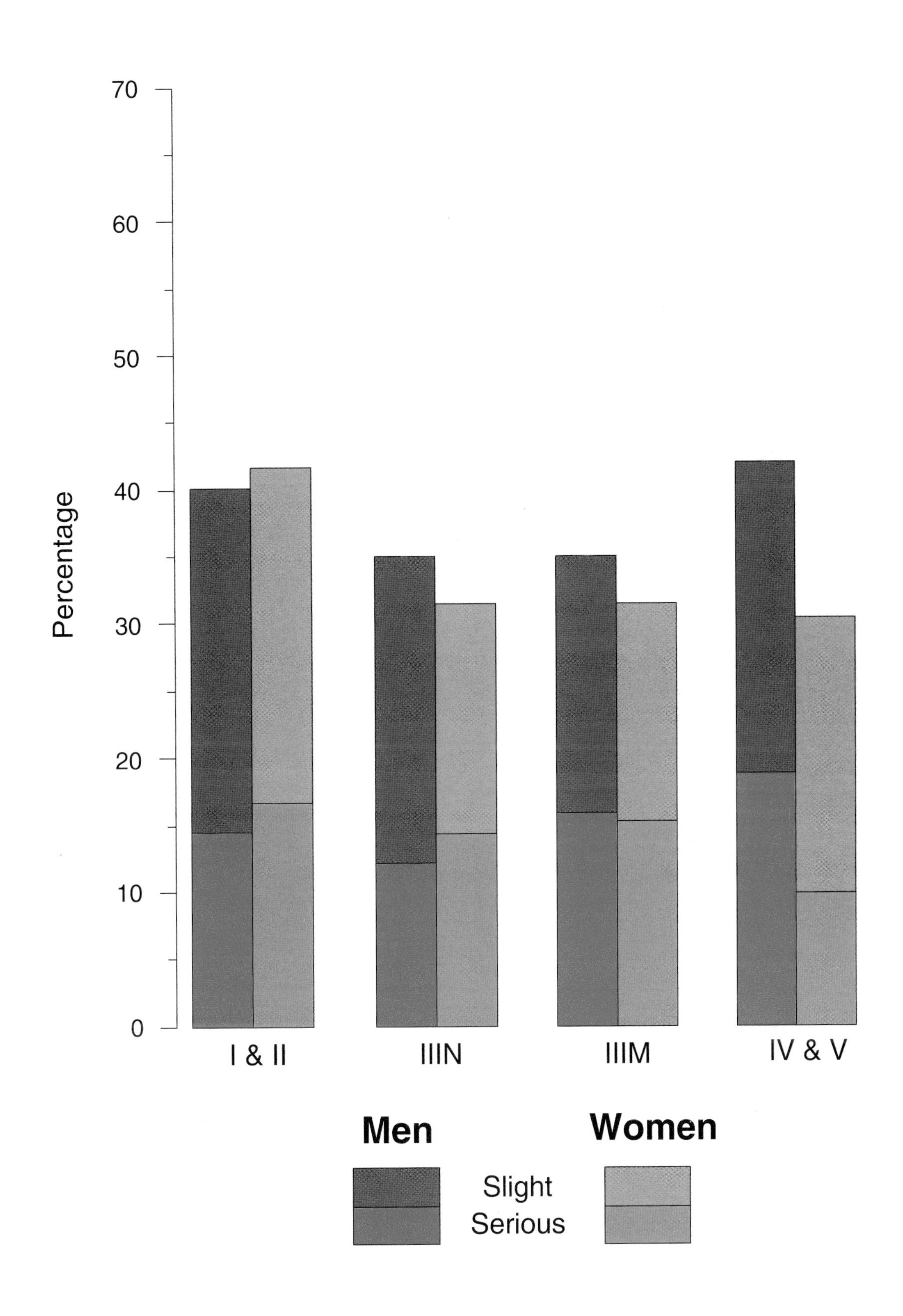

† Experienced in the past 12 months
Source: OPCS Omnibus Survey

Figure SB3: Prevalence of Sunburn†
by Marital Status & Sex Great Britain 1993

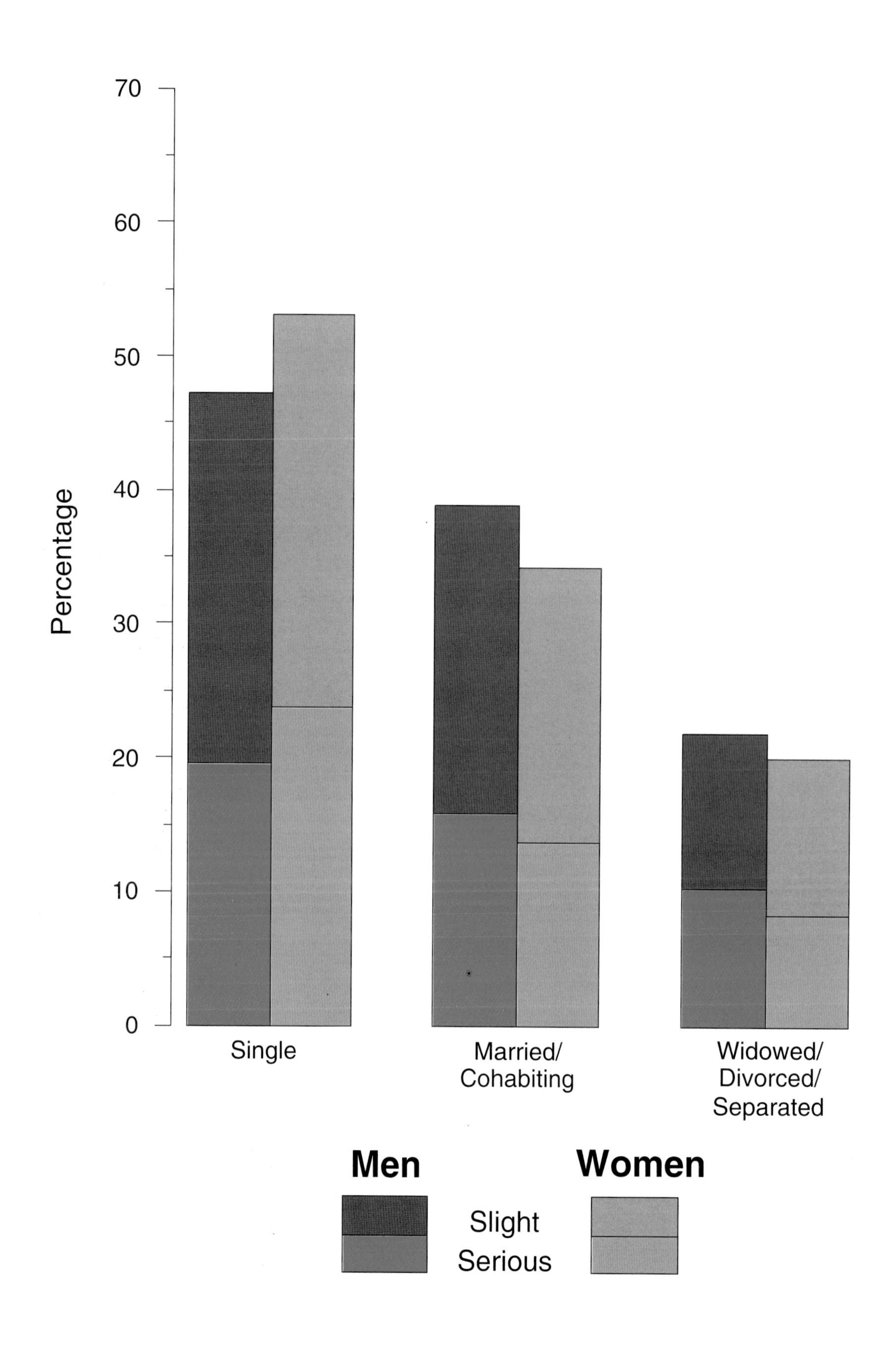

† Experienced in the past 12 months
Source: OPCS Omnibus Survey

Figure SB4: Prevalence of Sunburn†
by Household Type & Sex Great Britain 1993

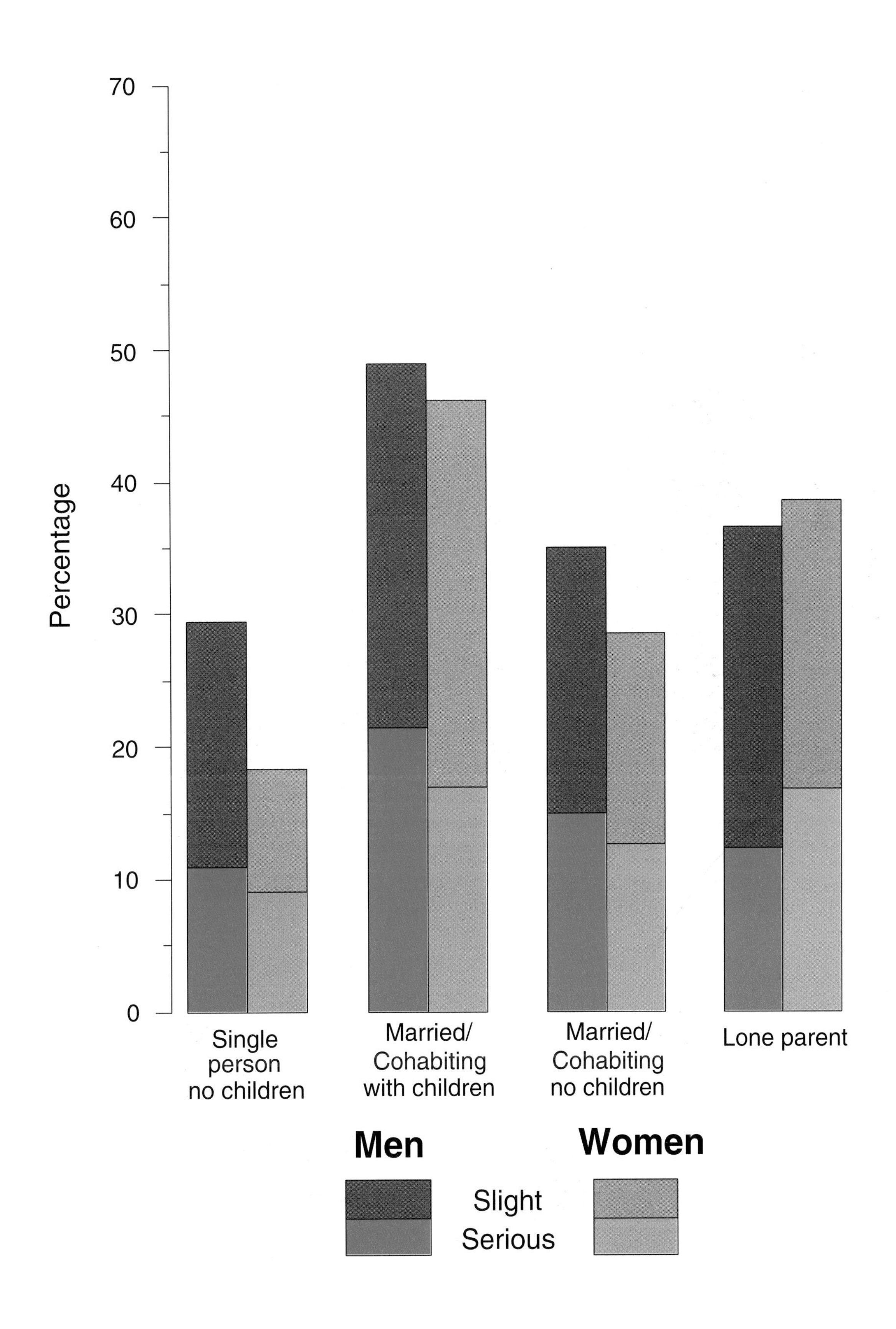

† Experienced in the past 12 months
Source: OPCS Omnibus Survey

SUICIDE

HON Targets:

to reduce the overall suicide rate by at least 15% by the year 2000 (from 11.1 per 100,000 population in 1990 to no more than 9.4)

to reduce the suicide rate of severely mentally ill people by at least 33% by the year 2000 (from the estimate of 15% in 1990 to no more than 10%)

The targets for suicide refer to specific self inflicted harm leading to death. Overall suicide rates are monitored through the registration of deaths and figures are published annually. The target data include both official suicides and deaths from injuries of undetermined cause, since epidemiological studies have shown that "undetermined" deaths are in fact nearly all suicides. This method gives a truer picture of actual suicides and avoids the problem of coroner variation.

Work is underway to establish the routine collection of data on suicides in people with severe mental illness, by linking coroner records with psychiatric services data.

Although mortality from suicide is very significant, nevertheless the main focus of mental health care is to improve morbidity and disability, and so the first target in the mental illness key area is to improve the health and social functions of people with mental illness. Work to develop a valid and reliable scale to measure health and social functioning in a routine clinical context at each care programme review is now nearly complete.

The OPCS Survey of Psychiatric Morbidity in Great Britain is now issuing a series of reports on the prevalence of psychiatric illness, use of services, and associated risk factors (including alcohol and drug use). The overall prevalence of non-psychotic disorders was 16% and of psychoses was 0.4%.

Secular trends and variation with age and sex Suicide rates in men have always been substantially higher than in women. For example, in 1992 the rates per million population in England and Wales were 169 and 60 respectively (suicide and undetermined injuries combined).

Until recently, suicide rates for both sexes have also been much higher in the elderly than in the young, but the rates have been falling in the elderly since the war.

Furthermore, since the early 1970s rates in young men have started to rise. Therefore these relative relationships are now changing and suicide rates in younger men have started to exceed suicide rates in older men. For women, suicide rates are still higher in older women than in younger women. *Figures SU1–2*

Hospital Episode Statistics show that in 1992/93 there were 53,011 incidents of suicide or admissions for self inflicted injury. This figure underestimates the numbers of such events because external cause was recorded for only two thirds of the admissions. The total number of people with self inflicted injuries will be even higher with the inclusion of those who did not attend hospital.

Socio-economic variation In an analysis of the variation of suicides with social class, OPCS found that men in social classes II, III and IV had low to average proportional mortality ratios (PMR – see glossary) for suicide and those in social classes I and V had higher PMRs, that is, classes I and V were the groups with higher suicide rates. There are no figures for women.

Marital status The suicide rate among men aged 15–44 was lowest for those who were married (1989). Widowed and divorced men had higher rates than single men but this was mainly a result of the different age structure of the two groups. Analysis by age showed that, in general, in each ten year age group, apart from the 15–24 year olds, single, widowed and divorced men had suicide rates which were three times greater than those of married men. Among women it was also the widowed and divorced who had the highest rates. *Figure SU3*

Ethnic group Suicide rates varied with country of birth. In 1979–83 the rates among 20–69 year olds were higher than average among people born in the African Commonwealth countries and lower than average for those born in the Caribbean Commonwealth countries. Men from the Indian sub-continent had lower rates than average. *Table SU1*

Women born in the Indian sub-continent, overall, had average rates of suicide but the rate among young women is particularly high. Among those aged 15–24 born in the Indian sub-continent, the rate is nearly three times higher than average for the same age group in England and Wales as a whole.

Geographical variation There was some variation with region in the suicide rates of men and women. *Regional Tables in appendix*

References and notes

OPCS. Survey of Psychiatric Morbidity in Great Britain Report No. 1, HMSO 1995

OPCS. Population Trends no 69 Trends in suicide deaths in England and Wales London HMSO 1992

OPCS Population Trends no 71 Suicide deaths in England and Wales trends in factors associated with suicide deaths London HMSO 1993

OPCS Mortality Statistics Series DH2 no 19
OPCS Mortality Statistics Series DH5 no 18

Soni Raleigh V, Balarajan R. Suicide and self burning among Indians and West Indians in England and Wales. British Journal of Psychiatry 1992; 161 365–8

Soni Raleigh V, Bulusu L, Balarajan R. Suicides among immigrants from the Indian sub-continent. British Journal of Psychiatry 1990; 156 46–50

Figure SU1: Suicides & Undetermined Injuries
by Age & Sex England & Wales 1992

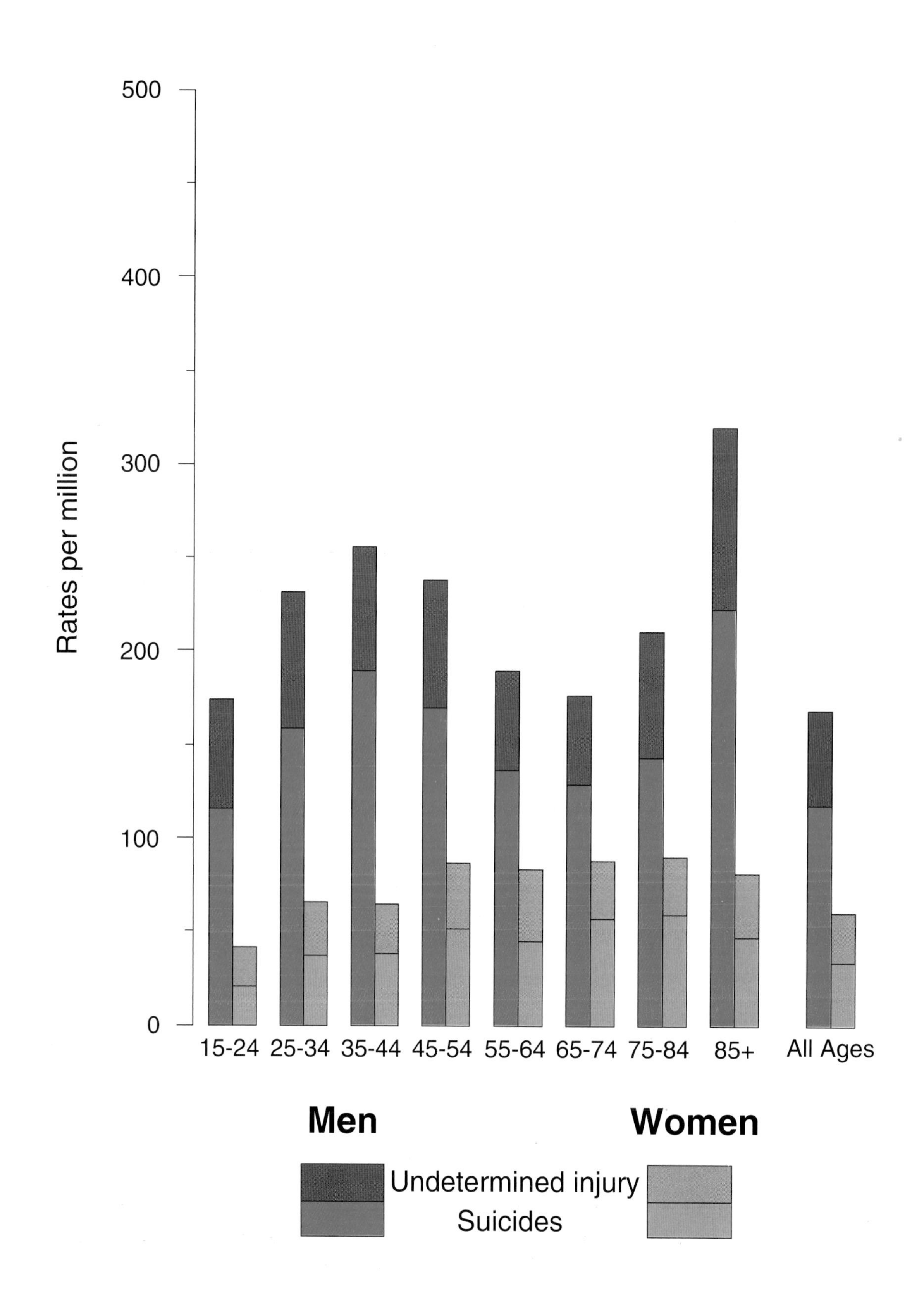

Source: OPCS Series DH2 no.19

Figure SU2: Suicide Rates per Million Population
by Age England & Wales 1946–1990

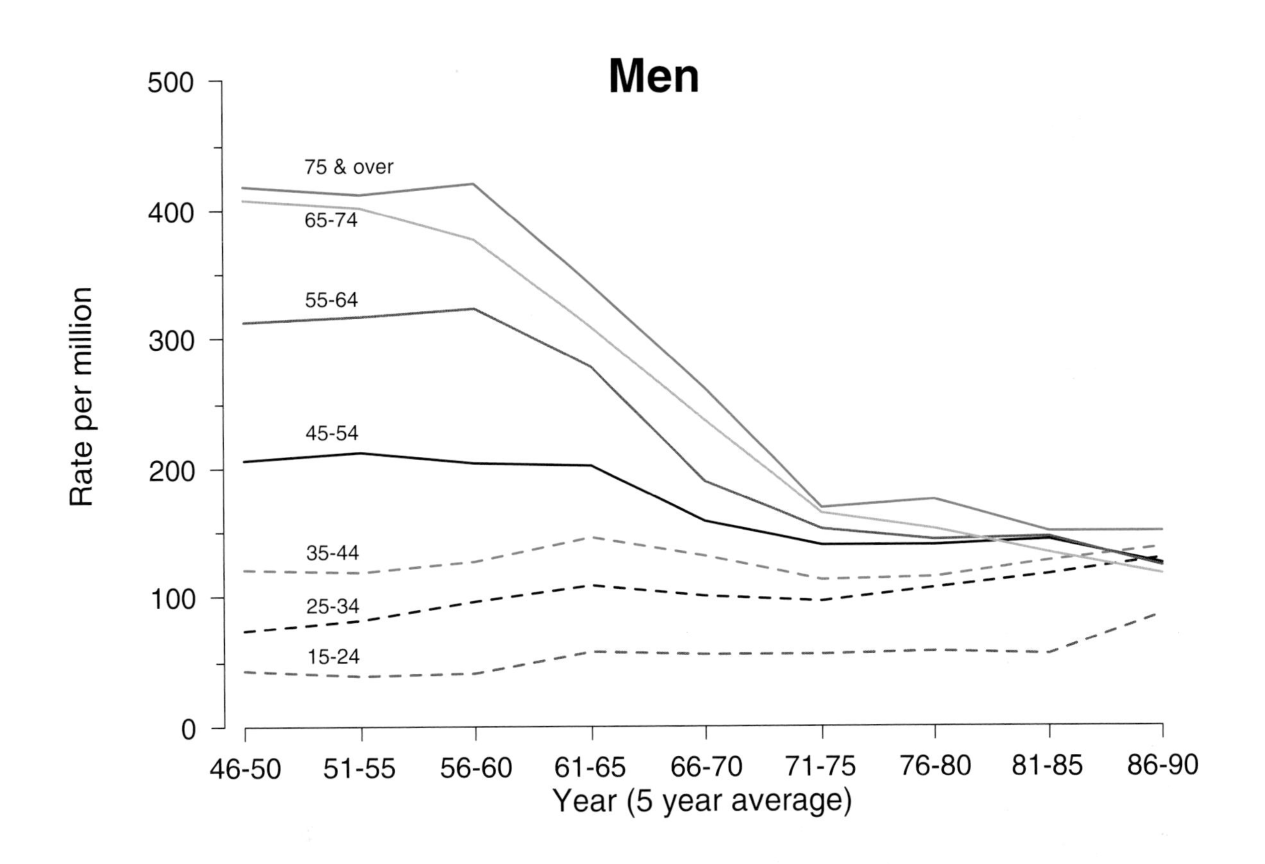

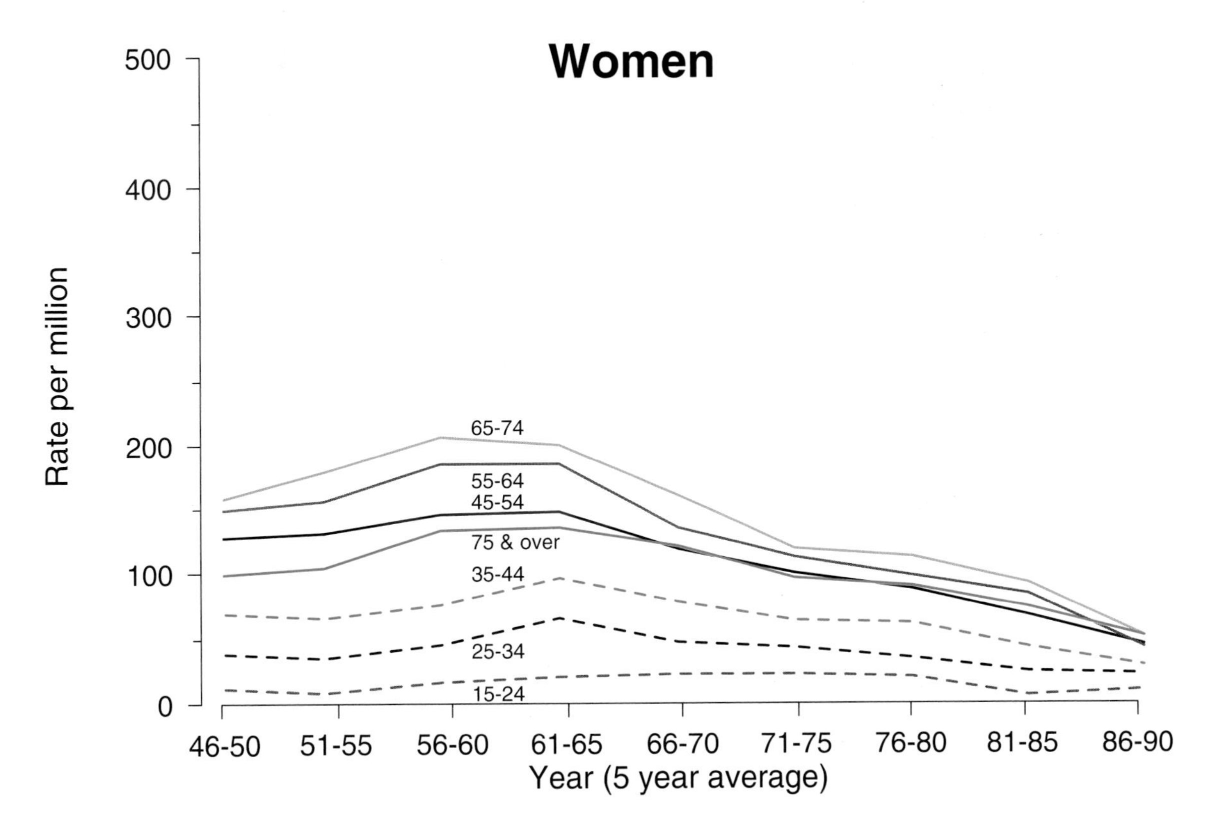

Source: OPCS Population Trends no. 69

Figure SU3: Suicide & Undetermined Injuries
by Marital Status & Sex, Age 15–44 England 1987–89

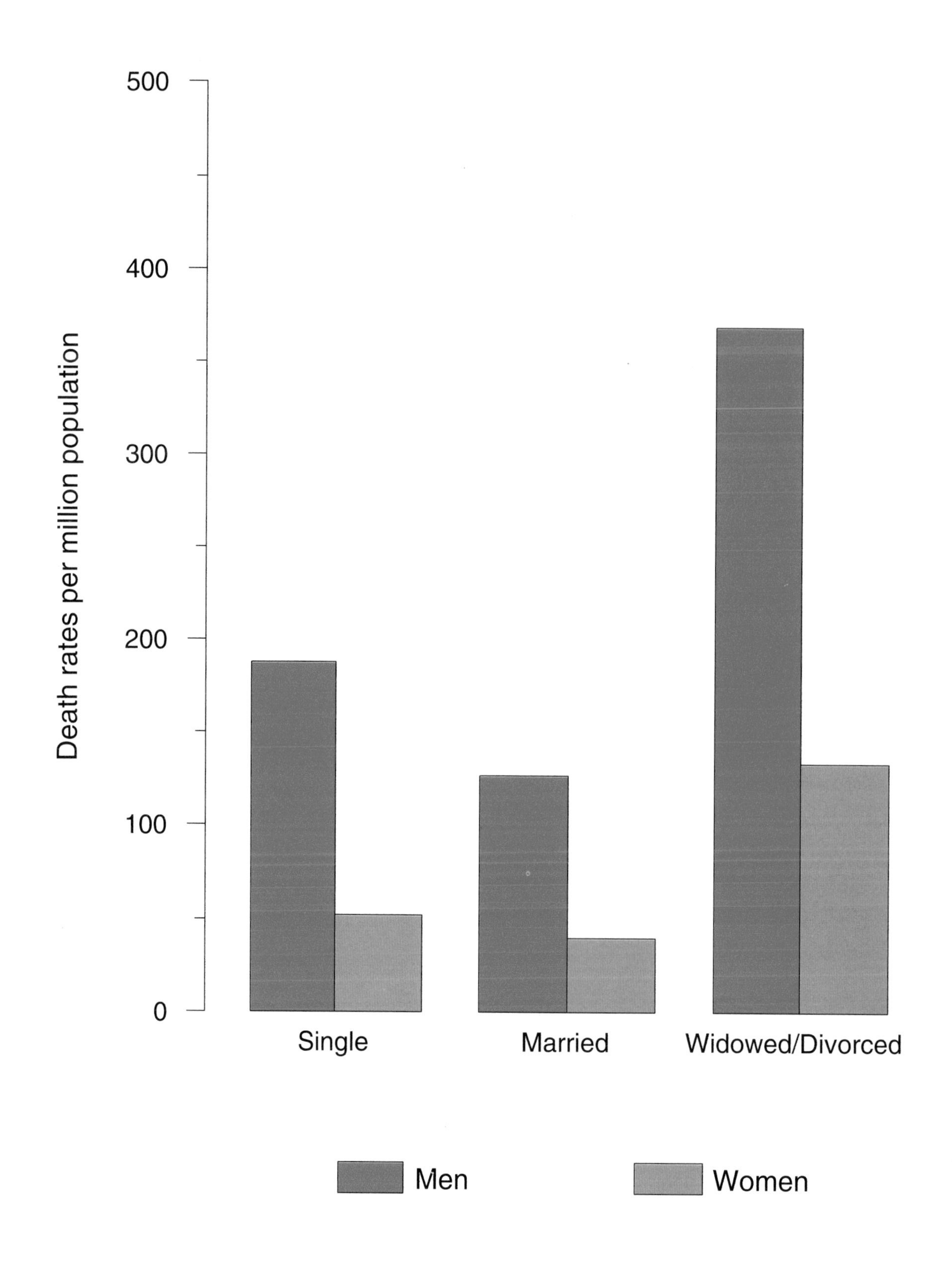

Source: OPCS Population Trends no.71

Table SU1 *Mortality from suicide by selected place of birth, England and Wales, 1979–83 (SMRs)*

	Age 20–49		**Age 20–69**	
Place of birth	**Men**	**Women**	**Men**	**Women**
Indian subcontinent	74	121	71	103
Caribbean Commonwealth	80	67	80	59
African Commonwealth	125	132	126	32

Standardised mortality ratios for England and Wales=100
Source: Raleigh and Balajaran (1992)

SEXUAL BEHAVIOUR

HON Targets:

to reduce the incidence of gonorrhoea among men and women aged 15–64 by at least 20% by 1995 (from 61 new cases per 100,000 population in 1990 to no more than 49 new cases per 100,000)

to reduce the rate of conceptions among the under 16s by at least 50% by the year 2000 (from 9.5 per 1,000 girls aged 13–15 in 1989 to no more than 4.8)

Gonorrhoea and other sexually transmitted diseases (STDs) are a major cause of ill-health and can have long term consequences. The target is useful as a proxy marker for behaviour which may also lead to HIV infection. Reducing the incidence of HIV infection is a Health of the Nation general objective but no specific targets were set because it was not possible to establish baseline rates of incidence and prevalence against which to measure future progress.

In 1994 the incidence of gonorrhoea was 37 cases per 100,000 population, a drop of 2% on the 1993 figure, clearly within the Health of the Nation target. The fall in incidence was slower than the successive falls of 24% and 17% in 1992 and 1993, indicating a levelling off of the downward trend. Overall, however, the gonorrhoea figure represents a significant improvement in sexual health and may have some relevance to reducing the transmission of other STDs including HIV infection.

Sexual behaviours which relate to these targets include contraceptive methods such as the use of condoms, the number of sexual partners and the age at first intercourse. These are also behaviours which relate to cervical cancer. Contraceptive methods other than the use of condoms are equally important in achieving the unwanted pregnancy targets.

Heterosexual behaviour

Secular trends and variation with age and sex Women aged 16–24 in 1990 experienced first sexual intercourse some four years earlier than had those aged 55–59 in 1990 (17 years compared with 21 years). This trend was also found among men.
Table SE1

14% of men aged 16–59 reported two or more heterosexual partners in the past year compared with 7% of women. The difference between the sexes in lifetime experience was even greater with 24% of men reporting ten or more partners compared with 7% of women. The proportion of both men and women reporting ten or more partners was highest among the 25–34 year olds.
Figures SE1/2

Among men and women with a heterosexual partner, 37% of men and 26% of women reported having used a condom at some time in the past year. Condom use declined with age and more men than women in each age group reported using condoms. For example, among 16–24 year olds 61% of men and 42% of women with a heterosexual partner reported using a condom. *Figure SE3*

Condom use as reported by women aged 16 to 49 increased from 13% of all women in this age group in 1986 to 16% in 1991. This increase was apparent in all age groups under 30 and highest among those aged 18–19 (from 5% to 15%).

Socio-economic variation Median age at first intercourse was higher among the non-manual social class groups than among the manual and this was so for each age group. For example, among women aged 25–34 in social class I the median age was 18 compared with 16 among those in social class V. (Data not shown for other age groups.) *Figure SE4*

The proportion of people reporting two or more partners in the past year varied with social class but without an overall pattern. *Figure SE5*

Men in social class V were the most likely to have used a condom with a heterosexual partner in the past year (56%). This was also true of women although the differences were smaller. With the exception of this difference there was no general pattern with respect to social class. *Figure SE6*

Marital status Around 30% of single and of widowed, separated or divorced men reported two or more heterosexual partners in the past year which was considerably higher than the 4% of married men. 17% of single women and 11% of widowed, separated or divorced women reported two or more partners in the past year. *Figure SE7*

Among people with a heterosexual partner in the past year, 64% of single men and 47% of single women reported having used a condom compared with 28% of married men and 22% of married women. *Figure SE8*

Ethnic Group Among men, the median age at first intercourse was higher for Asian groups and lower for blacks, compared with whites, while for women there was no difference between the white and black median age. Overall, black and Asian women experienced first intercourse one year later on average than their male counterparts.

Under 16s conceptions Conceptions among the under 16s had been increasing but decreased slightly between 1990 and 1991. In 1991 the conception rate was 9.3 per 1000. *Figure SE9*

Research into teenage pregnancy shows that teenage mothers are more likely to come from lower socio-economic groups. This is backed up by data from OPCS on all live births within *marriage,* where socio-economic group is classified by occupation of the father. This shows that in England and Wales in 1992, the percentage of births to mothers aged under 20 was highest in the lowest social classes, and lowest in the highest social classes. The percentage of births to mothers aged under 20 in social classes IV and V combined was more than 5 times higher than in classes I and II combined. Conversely, the percentage of mothers aged 30 or over in the highest social classes was nearly one and a half times that in the lowest.

Conception rates tended to be slightly higher in the north of England and ranged from 5.7 in the South West Thames region to 12.9 in the Northern region.

Figure SE10

Homosexual behaviour

Among men aged 16–59, 4% said they had ever had a homosexual partner and 1% reported having had a same gender sexual partner in the past year. The equivalent figures for women were 2% and less than 1%. Men aged 25–34 were the most likely to have had a male sexual partner in the past year (1.5%).

There were large regional variations in the numbers of men reporting homosexual experiences. Most striking was the concentration of those reporting homosexual experience in London. More than twice the proportion of men reporting a history of same-gender experience and current practice lived in London than anywhere else in Britain.

With the exception of region, homosexual behaviour was reported across a broad range of social and demographic backgrounds.

Among men who reported ever having any same-gender sexual contact, 62% had no partner in the past 5 years and 16% had one partner. At the other end of the scale, 4% had 20 or more partners in the past 5 years and 1% had 100 or more partners.

References and notes

Wellings K, Field J, Johnson A, Wadsworth J. Sexual Behaviour in Britain Penguin Books 1994. An interview survey with self-completion booklet of over 18,000 adults aged 16–59 in 1990/91 in Britain.

OPCS General Household Survey 1991 London HMSO 1993 (Series GHS no 22)

OPCS Conception Series FM1 no 21

Table SE1 *Median age at first heterosexual intercourse by age and sex GB 1990*

Age	16–19	20–24	25–29	30–34	35–39	40–44	45–49	50–54	55–59
Men	17	17	17	17	18	18	18	19	20
Women	17	17	18	18	18	19	19	20	21
Base	*551*	*924*	*1,212*	*1,128*	*1,076*	*1,035*	*779*	*646*	*629*
	704	*1,163*	*1,673*	*1,563*	*1,355*	*1,214*	*971*	*972*	*994*

Source: Wellcome Trust The National Survey of Sexual Attitudes and Lifestyle

Figure SE1: Two or more Heterosexual Partners in the Past Year
by Age & Sex Great Britain 1990

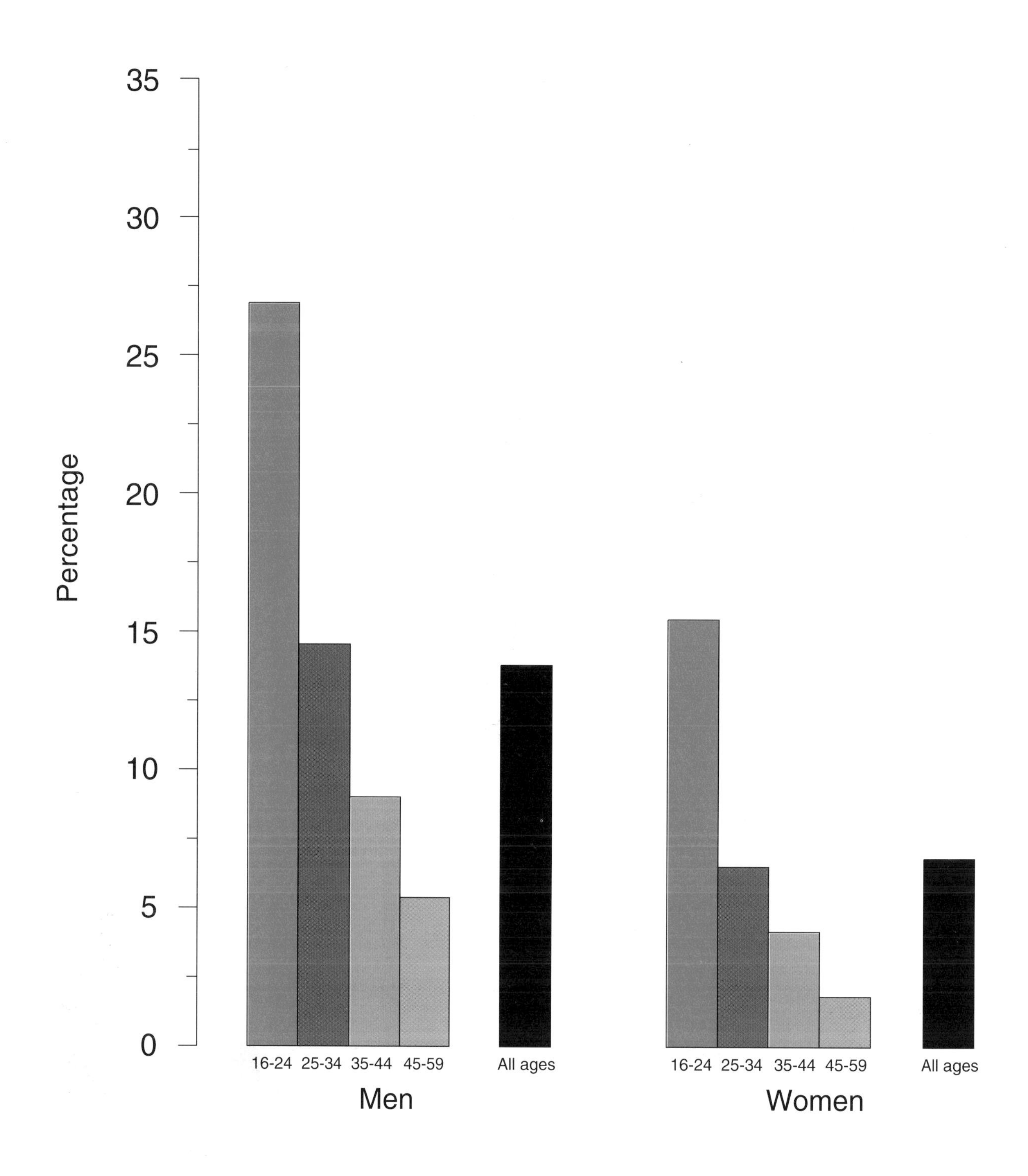

Source: Wellcome Trust National Survey of Sexual Attitudes & Lifestyle

Figure SE2: Ten or more Heterosexual Partners in Lifetime
by Age & Sex Great Britain 1990

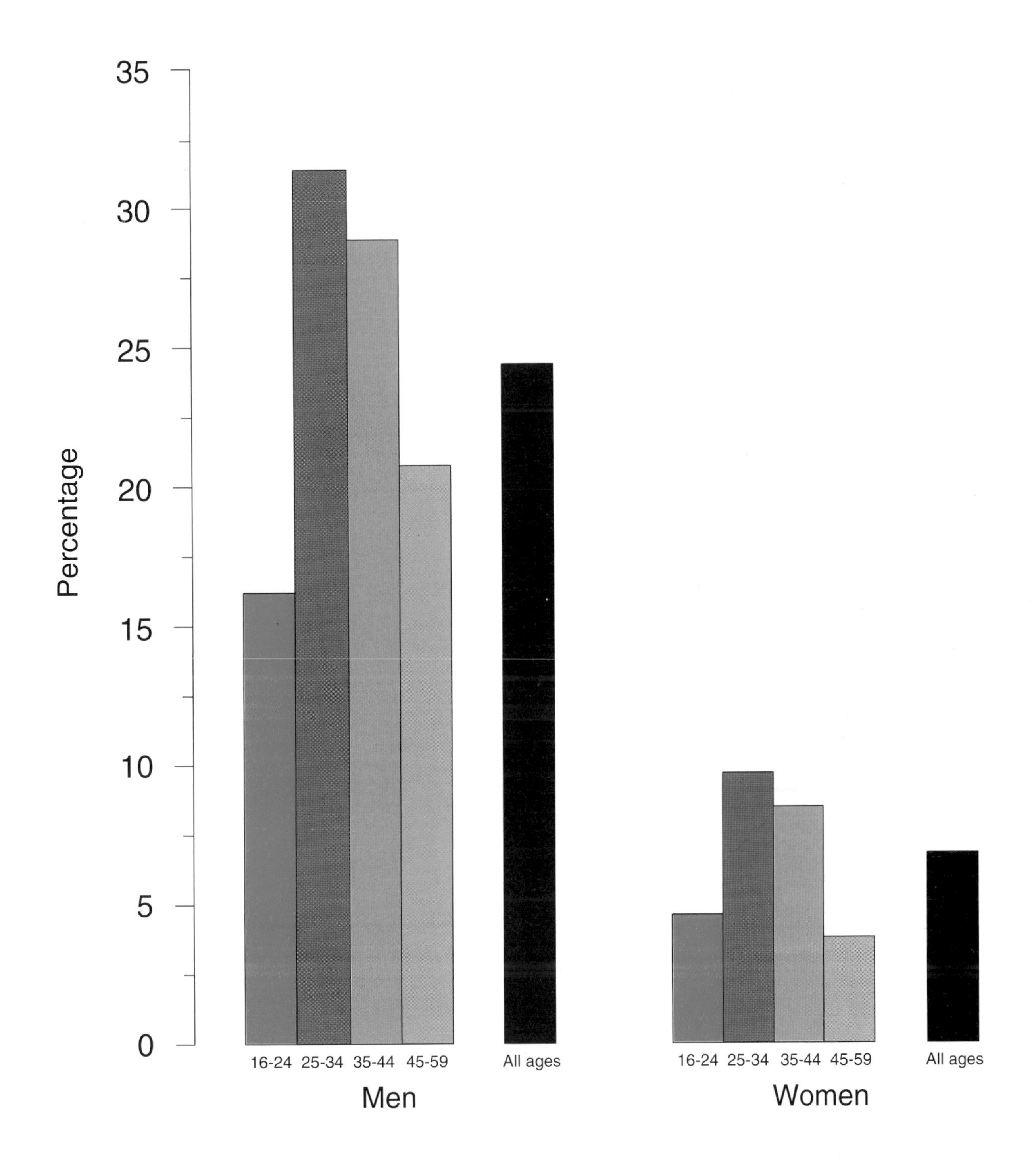

Source: Wellcome Trust National Survey of Sexual Attitudes & Lifestyle

Figure SE3: Use of Condoms in Past Year
by Age & Sex Great Britain 1990

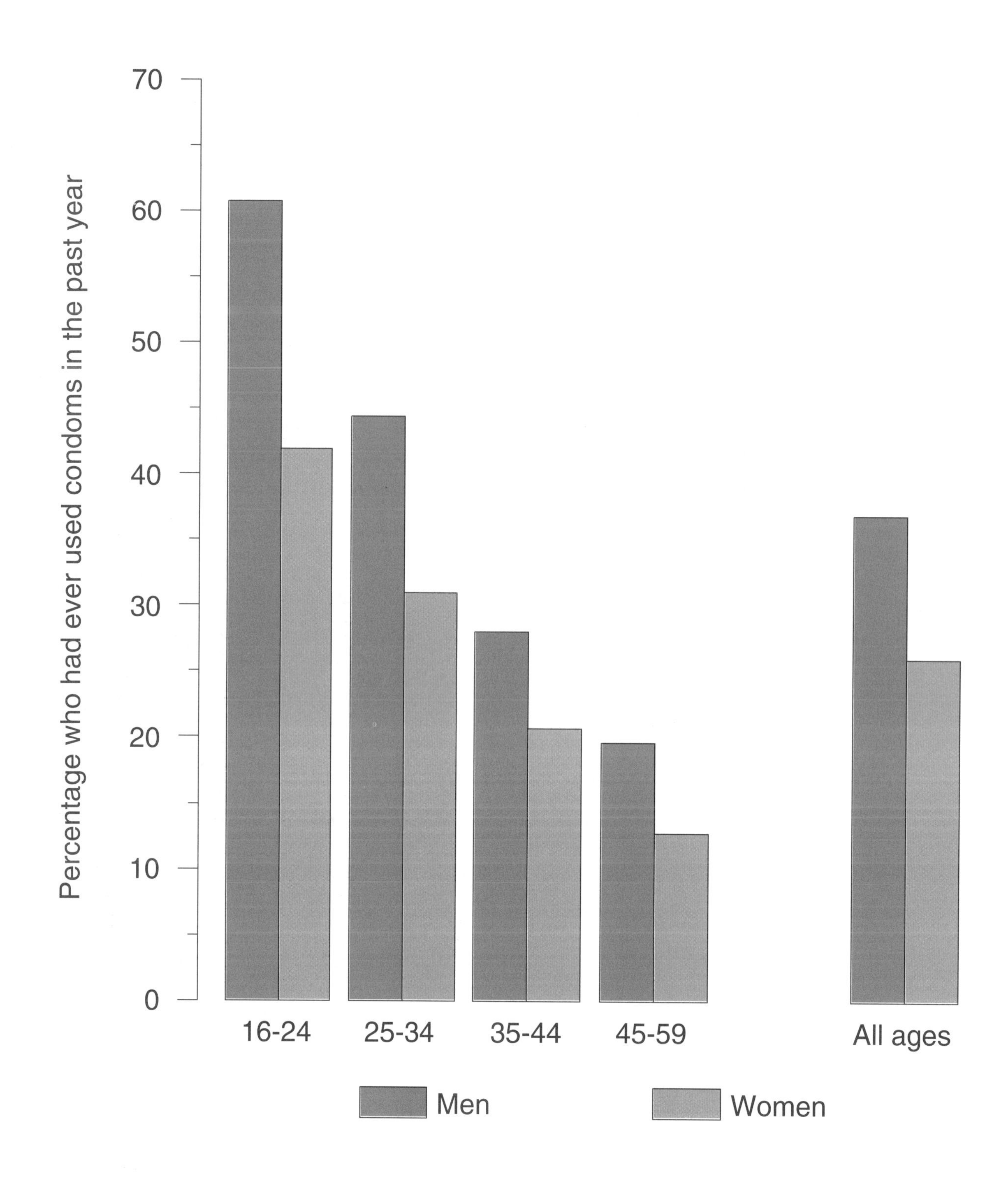

Excludes respondents with no heterosexual partners in the last year
Source: Wellcome Trust National Survey of Sexual Attitudes & Lifestyle

Figure SE4: Median Age at first Heterosexual Intercourse
by Social Class Great Britain 1990

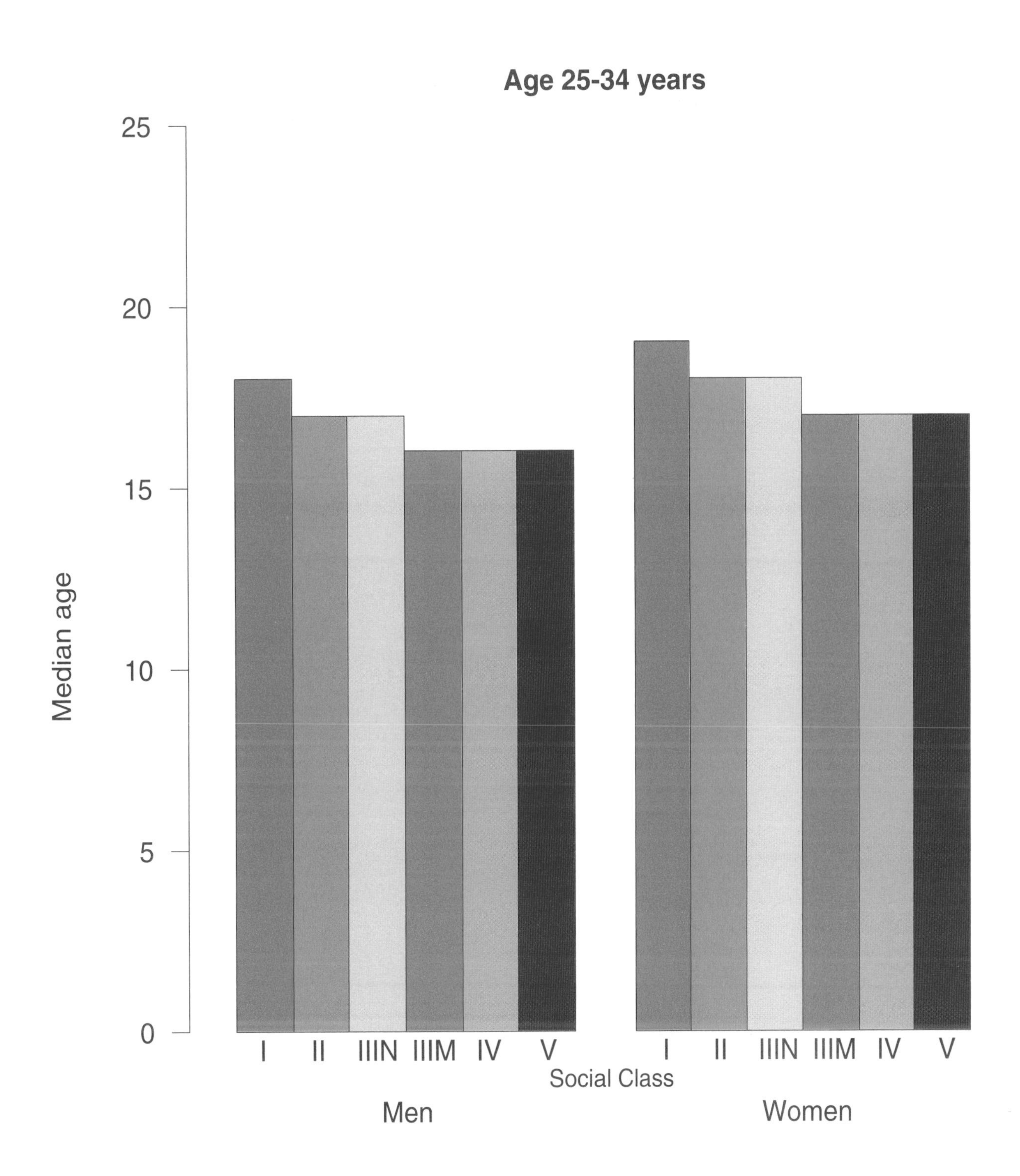

Source: Wellcome Trust National Survey of Sexual Attitudes & Lifestyle

Figure SE5: Two or more Heterosexual Partners in the Past Year
by Age, Sex & Social Class Great Britain 1990

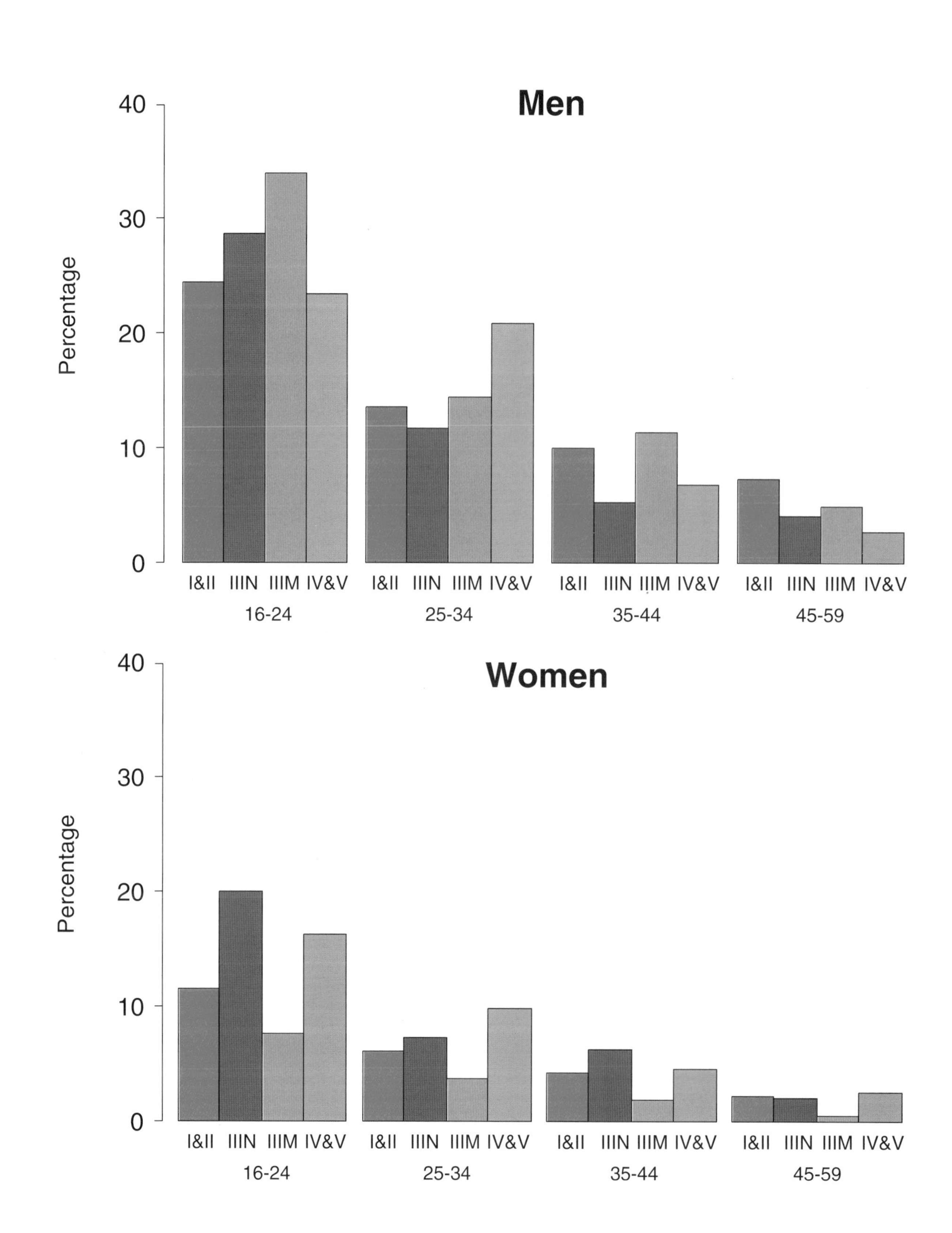

Source: Wellcome Trust National Survey of Sexual Attitudes & Lifestyle

Figure SE6: **Use of Condoms in Past Year**
by Sex & Social Class Age 16–59 Great Britain 1990

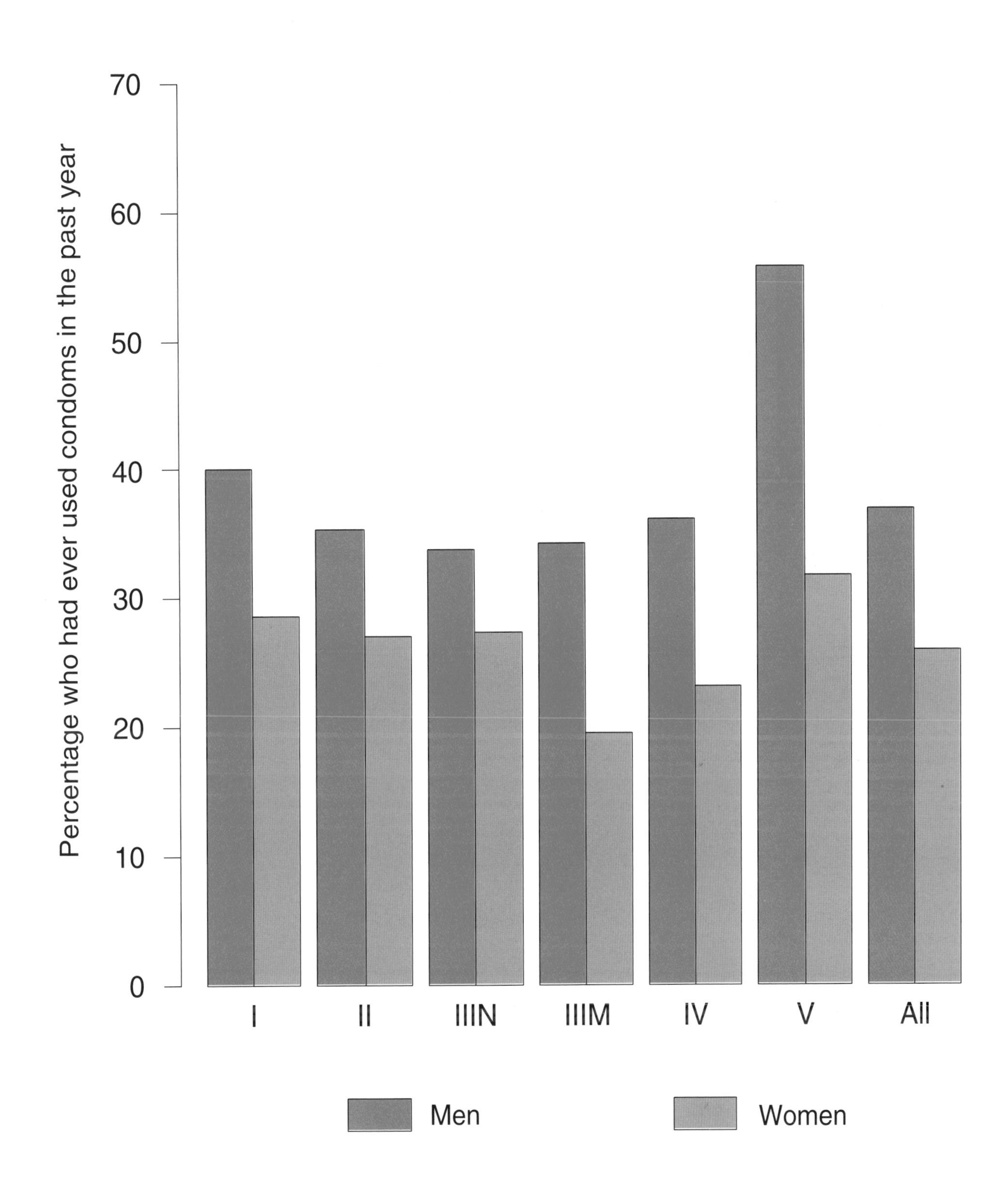

Excludes respondents with no heterosexual partners in the last year
Source: Wellcome Trust National Survey of Sexual Attitudes & Lifestyle

Figure SE7: Two or more Heterosexual Partners in the Past Year
by Sex & Marital Status Age 16–59 Great Britain 1990

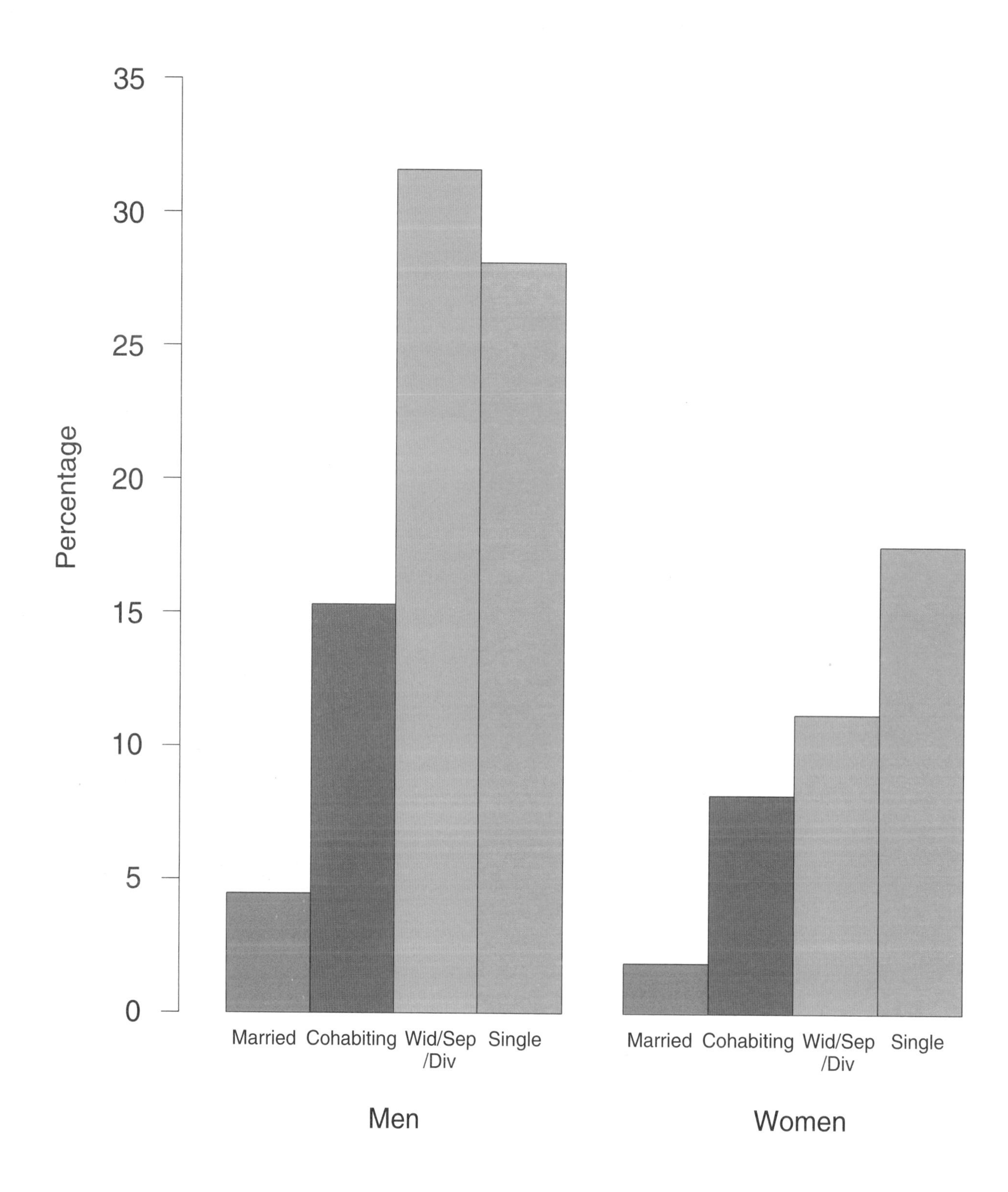

Source: Wellcome Trust National Survey of Sexual Attitudes & Lifestyle

Figure SE8: Use of Condoms in Past Year
by Sex & Marital Status Age 16–59 Great Britain 1990

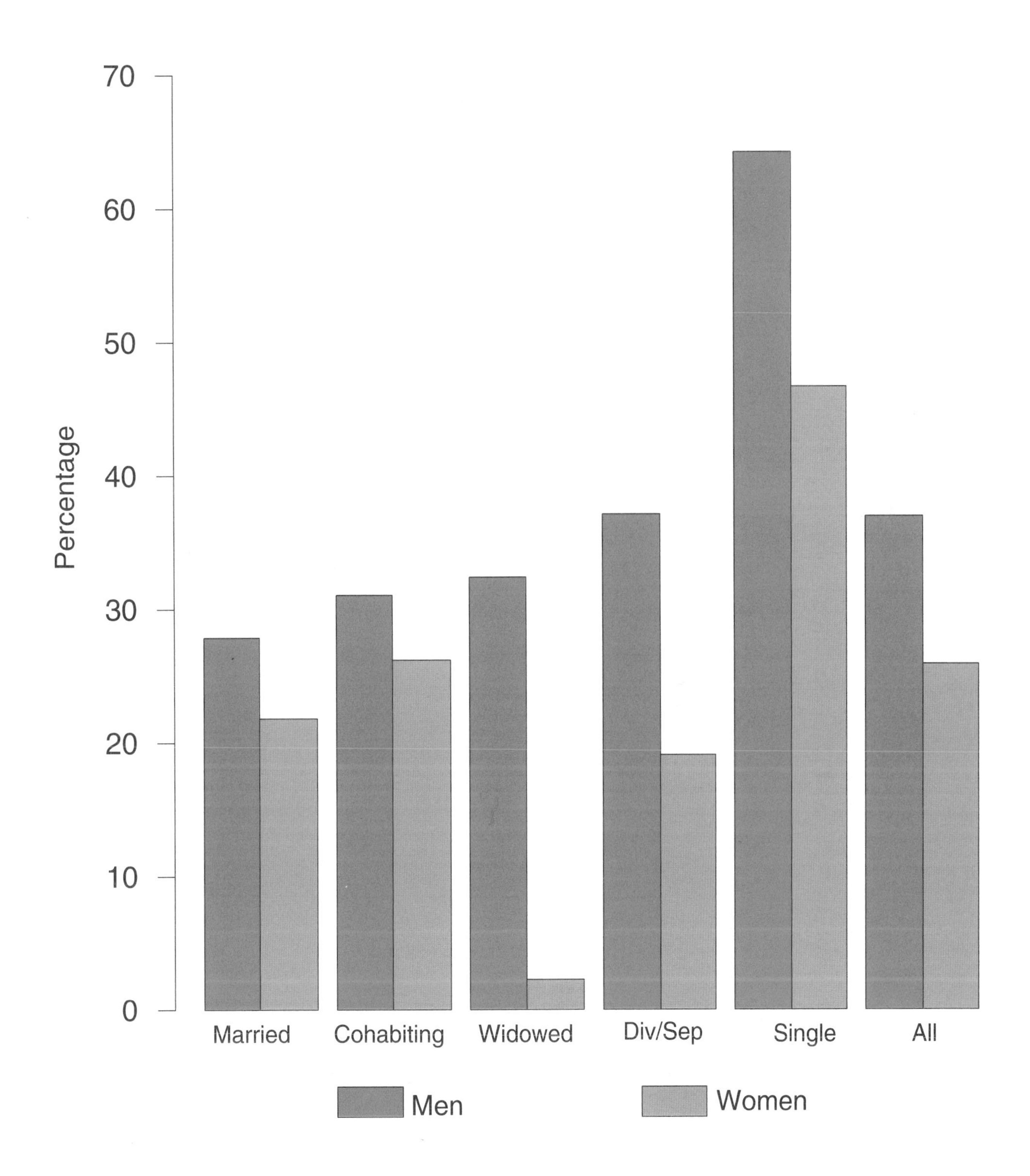

Excludes respondents with no heterosexual partners in the last year
Source: Wellcome Trust National Survey of Sexual Attitudes & Lifestyle

Figure SE9: Conception Rates per 1,000 Girls
Ages 13–15 England & Wales 1981–1991

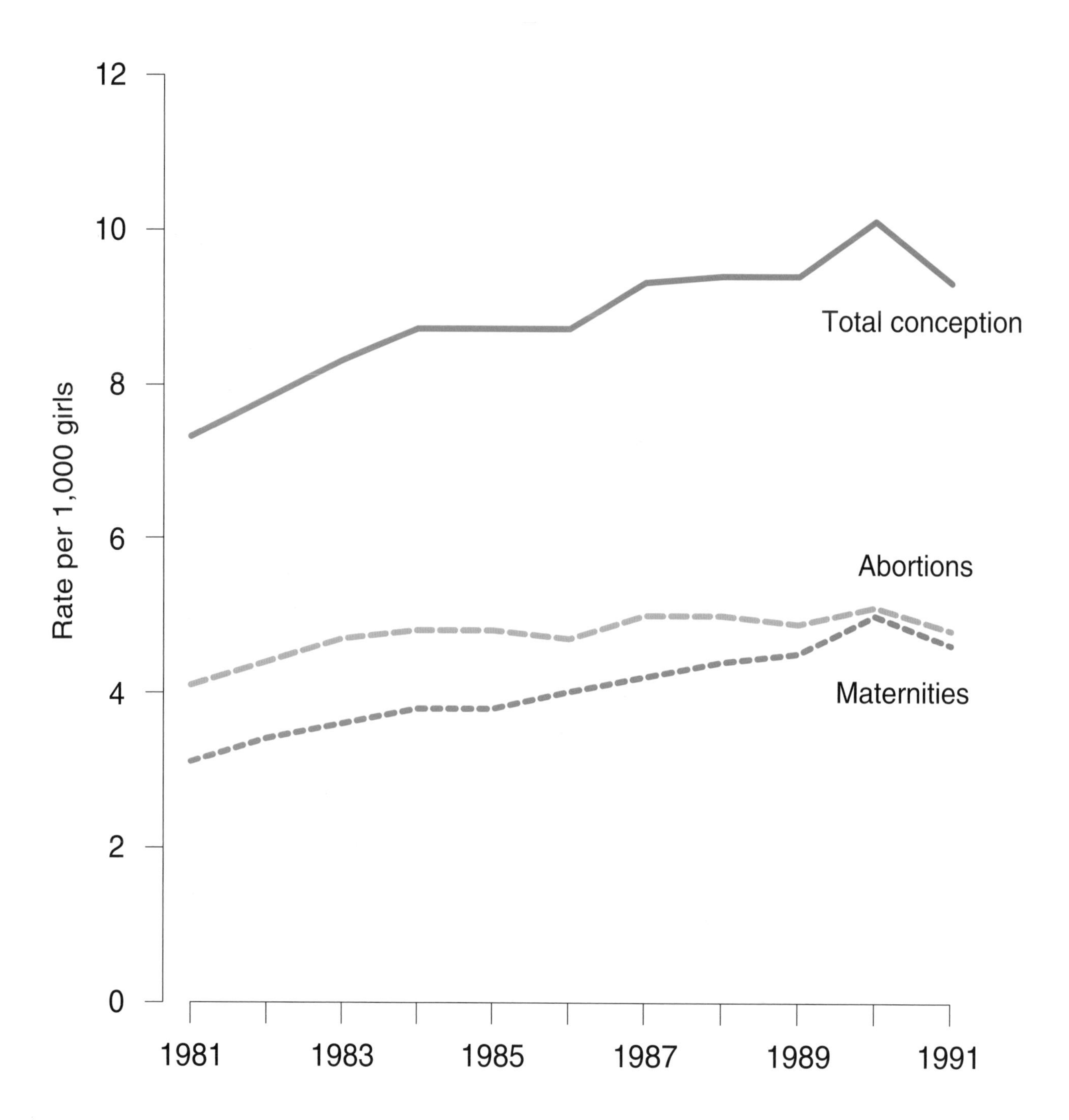

Source: OPCS Series FM1 no.21

Figure SE10: Conception Rates per 1,000 Girls
by RHA, Age 13–15 England 1991

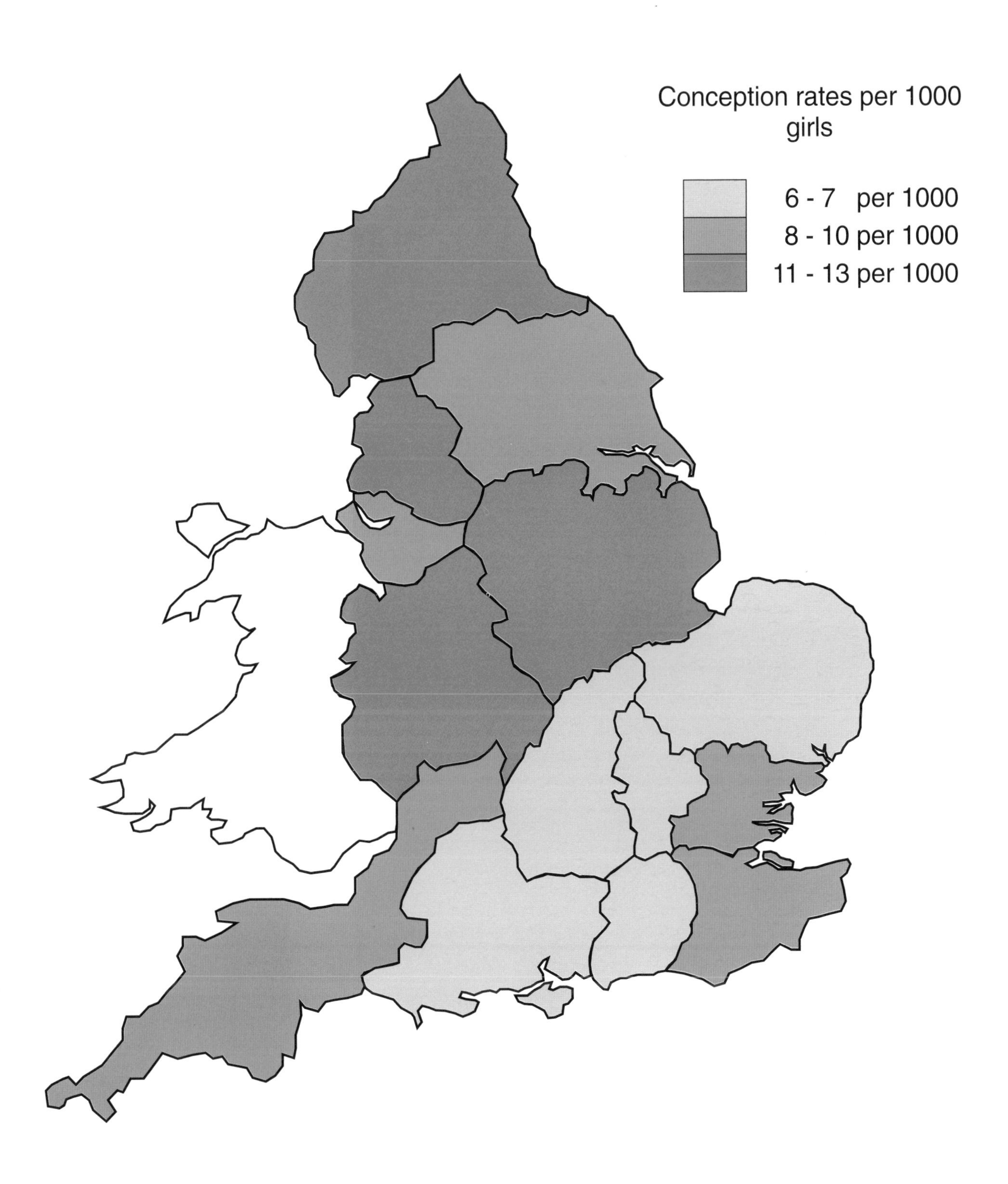

Source: OPCS Conception Series FM1 No.21

DRUG MISUSE

> HON Target:
>
> to reduce the percentage of injecting drug miusers who report sharing injecting equipment in the previous four weeks by at least 50% by 1997, and by a further 50% by the year 2000 (from 20% in 1990 to no more than 10% by 1997 and no more than 5% by the year 2000)

Anonymised surveys of groups of injecting drug misusers in London showed that, in 1993, between 4% and 7% were HIV positive. A reduction in the sharing of injection equipment will contribute to limiting the spread of HIV infection.

This target is a specific behaviour but there are no national figures. The main data available come from two multi-site studies, one based on attenders at syringe-exchange schemes and the other based on people in contact with selected drug treatment and advice centres including syringe-exchanges.

National figures will soon be available with the publication of a series of reports during 1995 from the OPCS Surveys of Psychiatric Morbidity in Great Britain. Information on injecting and sharing of equipment is also collected by the regional Drug Misuse Databases (DMDs). Although this information is not presently submitted to the Department of Health, discussion is currently in progress to determine the feasibility of doing so.

Secular trends The National Survey of Sexual Attitudes found that 0.4% of men and 0.2% of women aged 16 to 59 reported injecting non-prescribed drugs in the past five years. The first findings from the Survey of Psychiatric Morbidity (GB) suggest that the overall rate for drug dependence among people aged 16–64 was 22 per 1000 in the past year but figures on injecting drugs are not yet available.

Among attenders at 20 syringe exchanges in England and Scotland 21% reported sharing syringes in 1989/90 compared with 28% in 1987/88. Comparable data for non-attenders were 38% sharing in 1989/90 and 62% in 1987/88. *Figure DR1*

The unlinked anonymous HIV prevalence monitoring programme reports that in 1993, 17% of injecting drug misusers who were attending selected drug treatment and advice centres in London and the South East, reported injecting with used equipment in the past four weeks. The equivalent figure for the rest of England and Wales was 18% and, in 1992, 22% and 18% for the South East and the rest of the country respectively.

The study also reports that people aged less than 25 were more likely to share injecting equipment (25% compared with 14% of older injectors in the South East and 23% compared with 16% in the rest of England and Wales).

Socio-economic factors Donoghoe has reported that among attenders at syringe exchange schemes there were considerable levels of social disadvantage overall, but the sharers were more disadvantaged than the non-sharers. The sharers were less likely to support themselves with paid employment and more likely to live in unstable accommodation.

References and notes

Wellings K, Field J, Johnson A, Wadsworth J. Sexual Behaviour in Britain Penguin Books 1994.

OPCS. Survey of Psychiatric Morbidity in Great Britain Bulletin No. 1, OPCS 1994

Donoghoe M, Stimson G, Dolan K. Syringe Exchange in England An Overview, The Tufnell Press 1992. The data presented come from a study of people attending 20 syringe-exchanges. Although there is a higher proportion of non-attenders than attenders among injecting drug misusers, many attenders collect syringes for non-attenders as evidenced by the fall in syringe sharing among the non-attending group.

Department of Health, PHLS, Institute of Child Health. Unlinked Anonymous HIV Prevalence Monitoring Programme England and Wales. Department of Health 1995

Figure DR1: Syringe Sharing amongst Attenders & Non-attenders of Syringe Exchanges
England & Scotland 1987–90

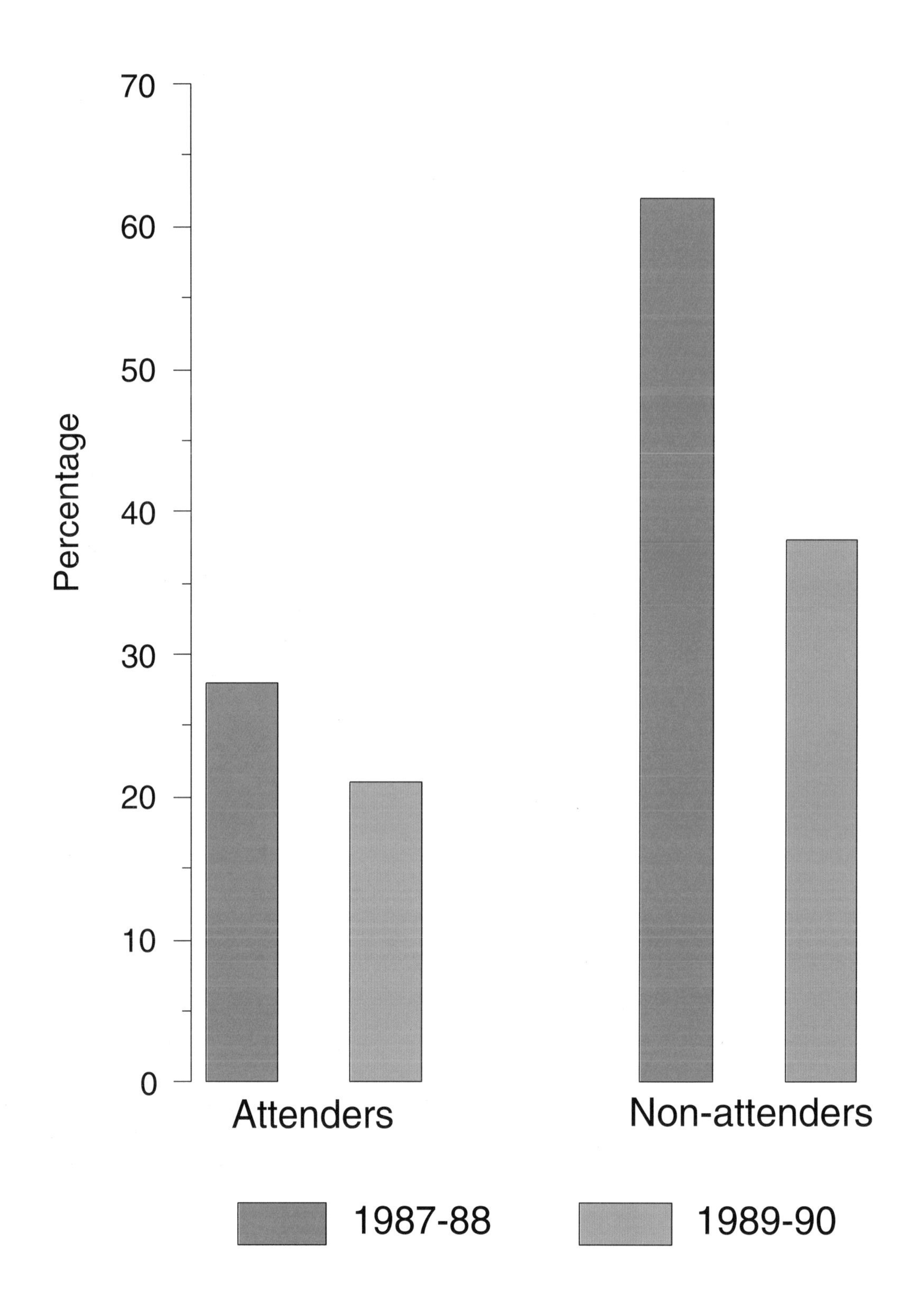

Source: Donoghoe: Syringe Exchange in England and Scotland

ACCIDENTS

HON Targets:

to reduce the death rate for accidents among children aged under 15 by at least 33% by 2005 (from 6.7 per 100,000 population in 1990 to no more than 4.5 per 100,000)

to reduce the death rate from accidents among young people aged 15–24 by at least 24% by 2005 (from 23.2 per 100,000 population to no more than 17.4 per 100,000)

to reduce the death rate for accidents among people aged 65 and over by at least 33% by 2005 (from 56.7 per 100,000 population in 1990 to no more than 38 per 100,000)

The three age groups defined in the targets are at risk from different types of accident. The under fives are most at risk from an accident in the home while up to the teenage years road accidents as a pedestrian are the largest cause of accidental death. Among 15–24 year olds, it is accidents as drivers or riders in vehicles that are the main cause of accidental death. Older people are at risk both in the home, from falls, and on the road.

Each type of accident has its own 'behaviours' but very few of these have been measured and many are dependent on external factors (for example the design of buildings). Many measures such as the use of seat belts or smoke alarms do not actually prevent accidents but reduce the severity of the outcome (which is relevant because the targets refer to reducing the *death* rate). Alcohol is a risk factor in accidents (see section on alcohol and road accidents) and fires caused by smoking are an important source of death and disability.

For this overview the death rates and numbers of casualties for different types of accidents are presented and one specific behaviour: the fitting of smoke alarms.

Overall variation with age and sex Accidental deaths accounted for 2% of all deaths in 1992 (England and Wales) but among young people under 25 this proportion was considerably higher, ranging from 12% for girls aged under 15 to 41% of 15–24 year old men.

Figure AC1

Although the proportion of deaths due to accidents was low among people aged 65 or more, the death rate per 100,000 population was higher than for the other age groups. For example in 1992 the death rates per 100,000 population for men and women aged 75–84 were 801 and 669 respectively compared with 313 and 91 for men and women aged 15–24. For each of the types of accidents presented in this overview, older people were more likely to die as the result of an accident than were younger people.

Among children aged under 15, road accidents accounted for about half of accidental deaths. Fire accounted for 20% of accidental deaths among girls and 14% among boys. For young men and women aged 15 to 24 the risk of death from road accidents far outweighed all other causes. Falls were the greatest cause of accidental death among people aged 65 and over. 65% of accidental deaths among women in this age group were as a result of falls. *Figures AC2(M) and (F)*

Ethnic group Death rates from fires and accidental poisonings were generally higher among people born in the Indian subcontinent, Caribbean and African Commonwealth countries. *Table AC1*

Geographical variation The standardised mortality ratios for the overall accidental death rate were generally lower in the south. The rates for motor vehicle deaths showed some variation with region ranging from 122 for women in East Anglia to 79 for women in the North East Thames region. There was more regional variation in respect of deaths from falls with SMRs ranging from 137 among men in the North West to 56 among men in Wessex and 55 among women in the South West Thames region. *Regional tables in appendix*

Road Accidents

The numbers of people killed or seriously injured in road accidents has decreased for all age groups since 1981–85 but the decrease in both the number of casualties and the overall casualty rate was much smaller. The overall casualty rate decreased most among children under 16 from 431 to 372 per 100 thousand population.

These decreases result from a combination of fewer accidents per 100 million vehicle kilometres and a gradual decrease in the proportion of accidents which cause fatal or serious injuries. *Table AC2*

The overall casualty rate was highest among 16–19 year olds. The majority of children under 12 who were killed in road accidents were pedestrians but from 16 to 29 the majority of deaths were among car users. The proportion of pedestrian deaths was also high among older people, in particular those aged 80 or more. The age grouping used in road accident statistics is different from those used in the target setting, so two age groups (25–29 and 60–64) are included in this Figure who are not included in the HON accident targets. *Figure AC3*

Comparison of the casualty figures with data from the National Travel Survey on 'exposure' to road accidents shows that the variation in casualty rates with age was not entirely due to different levels of exposure. For example, the casualty rate for car users was highest among 16–19 year olds but they travelled fewer miles on average per year than people aged 30–59. *Table AC3*

Fires

Between 1990 and 1993 in England and Wales fatalities in fires decreased from 15 to 11 people per million population but during this period the rate of non-fatal casualties increased slightly from 233 to 238 people per million population.

Figure AC4

It is estimated that 35% of fatalities and 20% of non-fatal casualties occurred in fires started by smokers' materials.

More men died or were injured in fires than women (17 and 272 compared with 11 and 192 fatal and non-fatal casualties per million population).

The death rate was highest among people aged 65 or more and lowest for those aged 5–16. The non-fatal casualty rate was also lowest for this age group. Data presented refer to HON accident target age groups. *Figure AC5*

Smoke alarms In 1992, 50% of homes in Great Britain had a smoke alarm. This proportion had increased significantly from 45% in 1991.

The combined data for the two years showed that households headed by someone aged 35–44 were the most likely to contain a smoke alarm and those headed by someone aged 75 or more the least likely (52% compared with 33% – see notes). *Figure AC6*

Smoke alarms – socio-economic status and household type There was no difference between the proportion of manual and non-manual households with a smoke alarm (44% of each – see notes).

Households comprising a married couple with dependent children were the most likely to have a smoke alarm (61%) but lone parents with dependent children were less likely to have an alarm (46%). Single person households and lone parents without dependent children were the least likely to have a smoke alarm (35% and 32%).

Smoke alarms – geographical variation Households in Scotland were the most likely to have a smoke alarm (60%), and those in the North, Midlands and East of England were the least likely to do so (44% and 43%).

HOME ACCIDENTS

Home accidents resulted in 3,986 deaths in England and Wales in 1992 and accounted for about 40% of all fatal accidents. The death rate for accidents in the home increased with age among adults but was higher among the under 5s than older children. Boys had a higher death rate than girls for accidents in the home and among adults the rate for men exceeded that for women except for people aged 75 or more. *Table AC4*

In 1987–89 1% of males and 2% of females were reported to have had an accident in the home in the past three months which resulted in them seeing a doctor or attending hospital. This proportion was 4% for children aged less than 5 and 3% for women aged 75 or more.

During 1992 in the UK it is estimated that about 2.55 million people were treated in hospital as a result of an accident at home. Falls were the most frequent reason for a home accident to result in attendance at an A&E department. Being cut or struck were two other frequent reasons.

The types of home accidents resulting in visits to A&E departments varied considerably with age. 65% of home accidents among people aged 65 or more were the result of falls compared with 30% of people aged 15–64. Being struck by or colliding with an object was most frequent among 5–14 year olds (23% of accidents). Falls were more common among the youngest age group, accounting for 46% of home accidents. *Figure AC7*

References and notes

OPCS Mortality Statistics Series DH2 no 19 E&W 1992
OPCS Mortality Statistics Series DH4 no 18 E&W 1991
OPCS Mortality Statistics Series DH5 no 18 E&W 1991

DoT Road Accidents Great Britain 1992 The Casualty Report
DoT Road Accidents Great Britain 1993 The Casualty Report

DoT National Travel Survey 91/93 London HMSO 1994

Home Office Statistical Bulletin – Summary Fire Statistics UK 1993 Issue 29/94
Home Office Fire Statistics UK 1992

OPCS National Fire Safety Week and Domestic Fire Safety London HMSO 1994
GB AGE 16+ The base for household data was all households interviewed in September 1991, November 1991, September 1992 and November 1992 (8,267 households). One adult per household was selected at random for interview. Details referring to the head of household (age and social class) were only ascertained where that individual was the head of household (5,040 individuals). These two different samples yield slightly different results.

DTI Home and Leisure Accident Research 1992 Data DTI 1994 UK All ages

OPCS General Household Survey 1989 London HMSO 1991 (Series GHS; no 20)

Balarajan R and Bulusu L Mortality among immigrants in England and Wales, 1979-83 in Mortality and Geography OPCS Series DS no. 9 London 1990

Figure AC1: Accidental Deaths as a percentage of all deaths
by Age & Sex England & Wales 1992

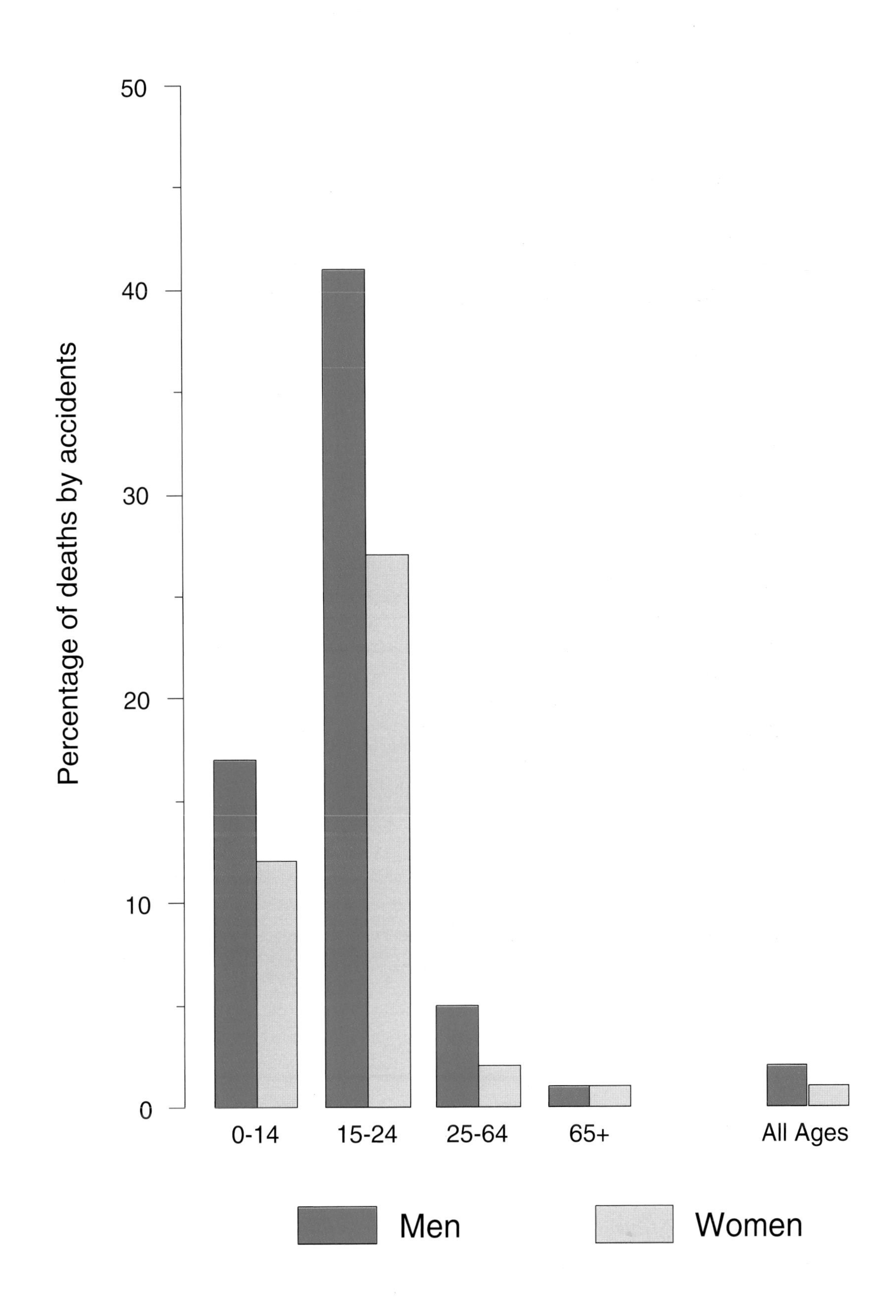

Source: OPCS Series DH2 no.19

Figure AC2(M): Accidental Deaths
by Type of Accident & Age England & Wales 1992

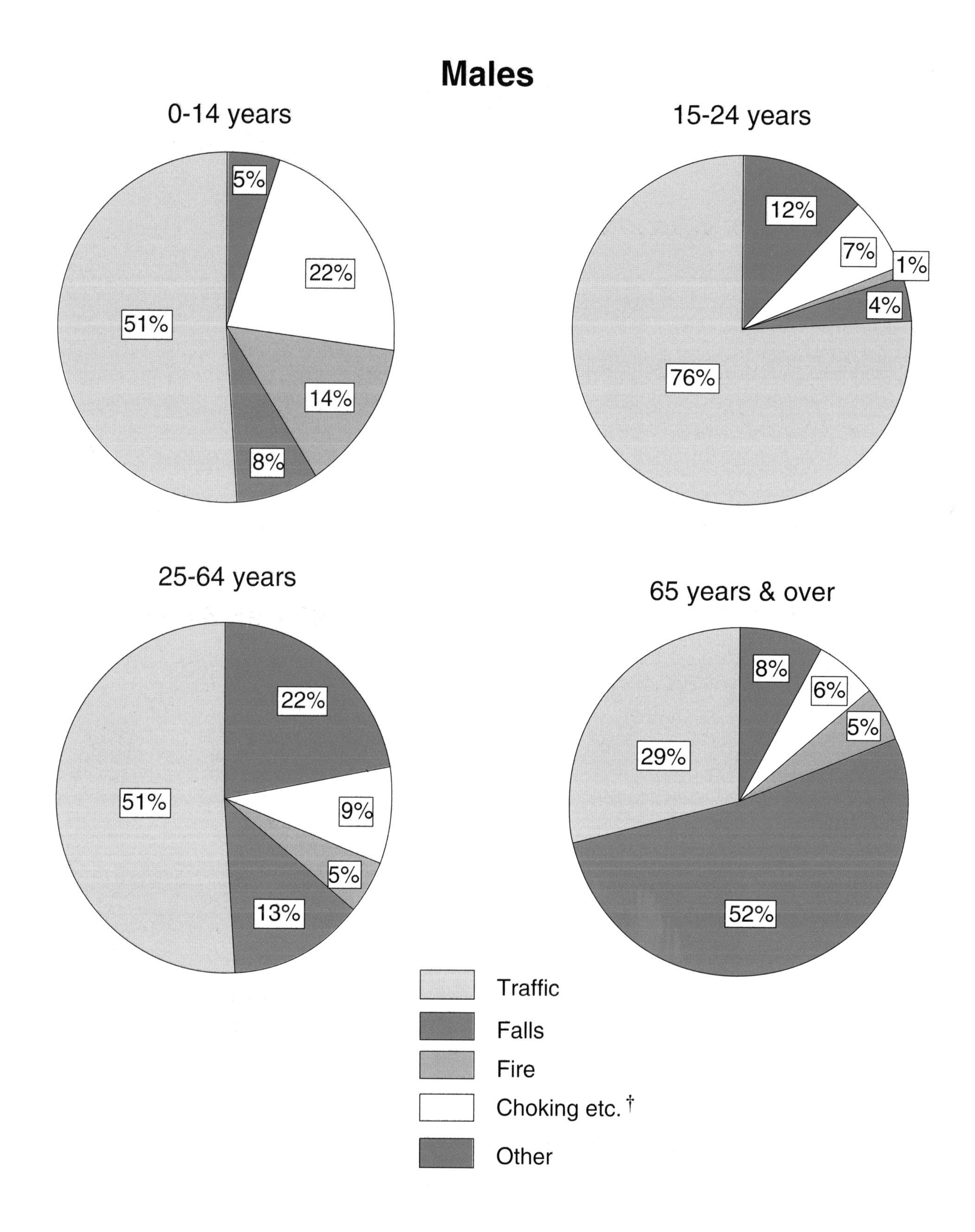

† Choking etc. includes death from submersion, suffocation and foreign bodies
Source: OPCS Series DH2 no.19

Figure AC2(F): Accidental Deaths
by Type of Accident & Age England & Wales 1992

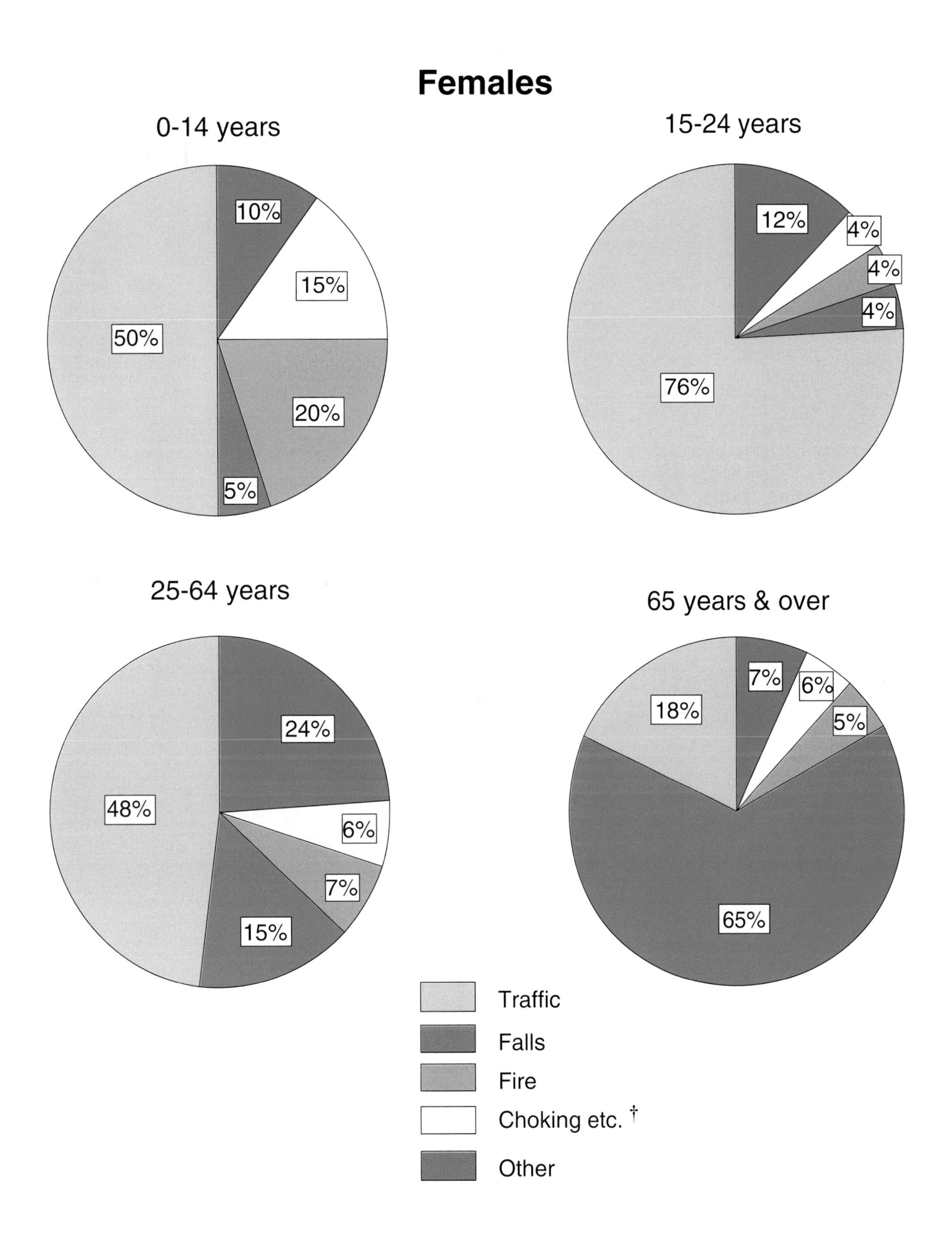

† Choking etc. includes death from submersion, suffocation and foreign bodies
Source: OPCS Series DH2 no.19

Figure AC3: Death & Casualty Rates† by Type of Road User
by Age Great Britain 1993

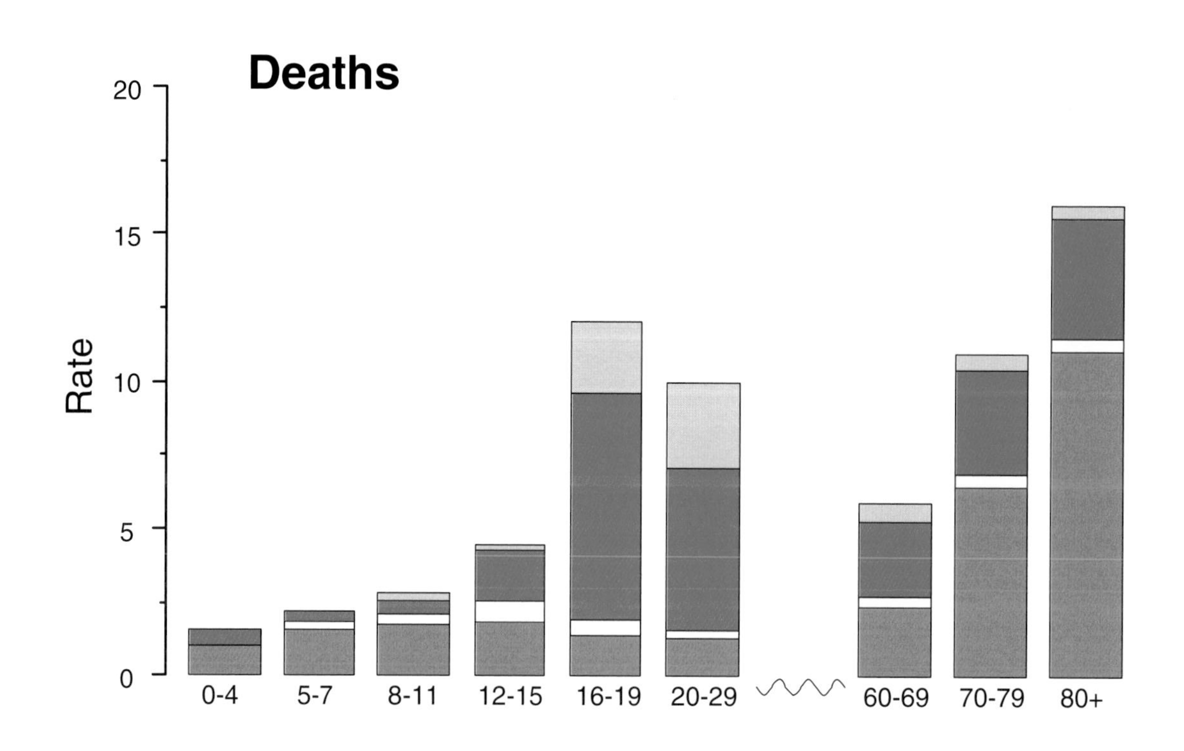

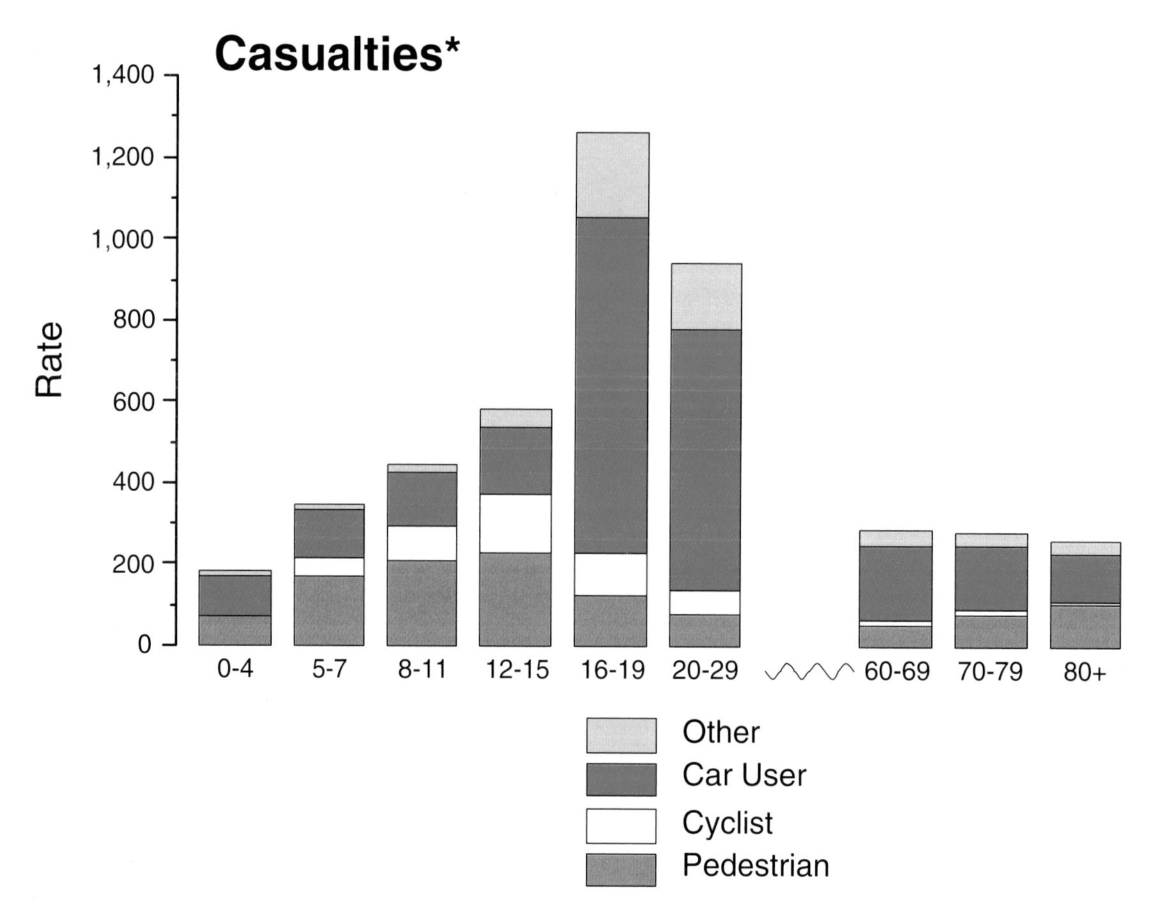

† Rate per 100,000 of population
* Casualties include fatalities
Source: DoT Road Accidents GB 1993 – The Casualty Report

Figure AC4: Casualties from Fires
All Ages England & Wales 1983–1993

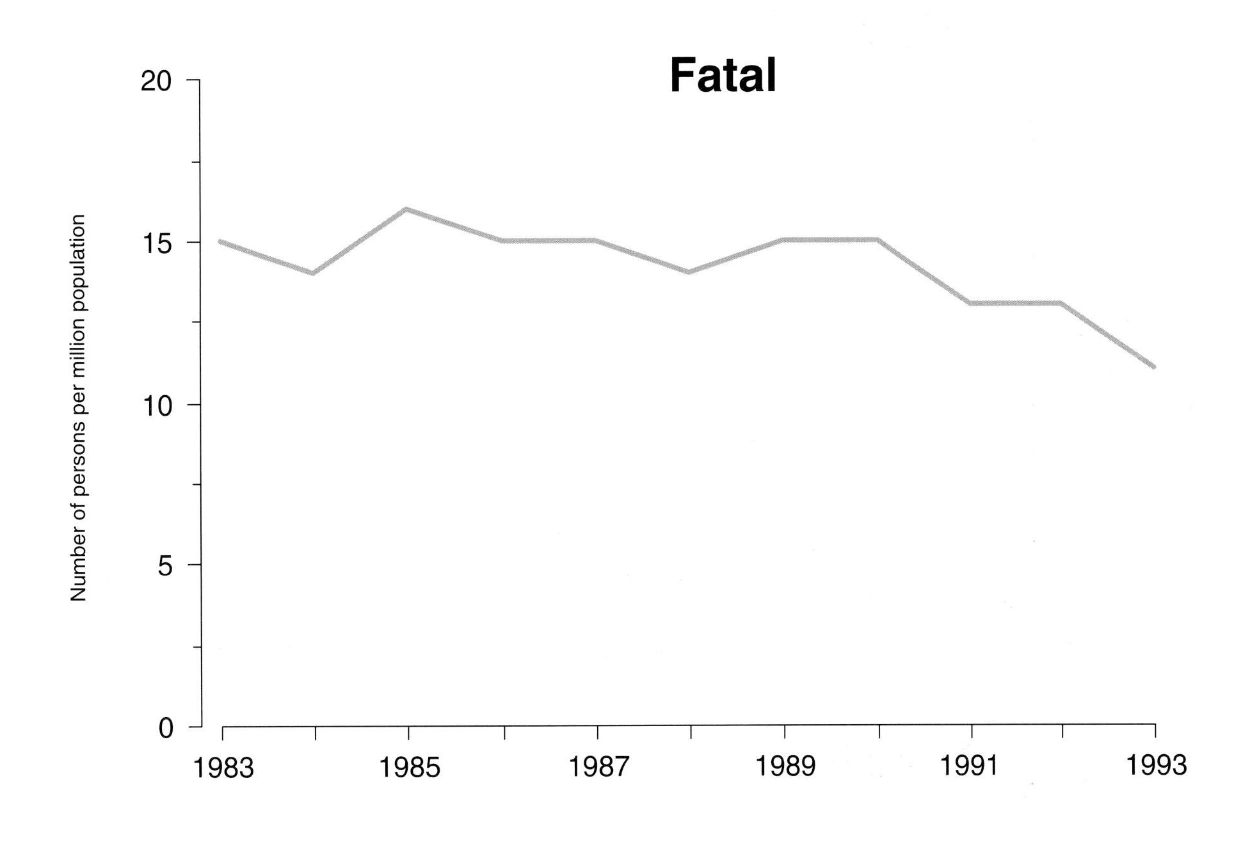

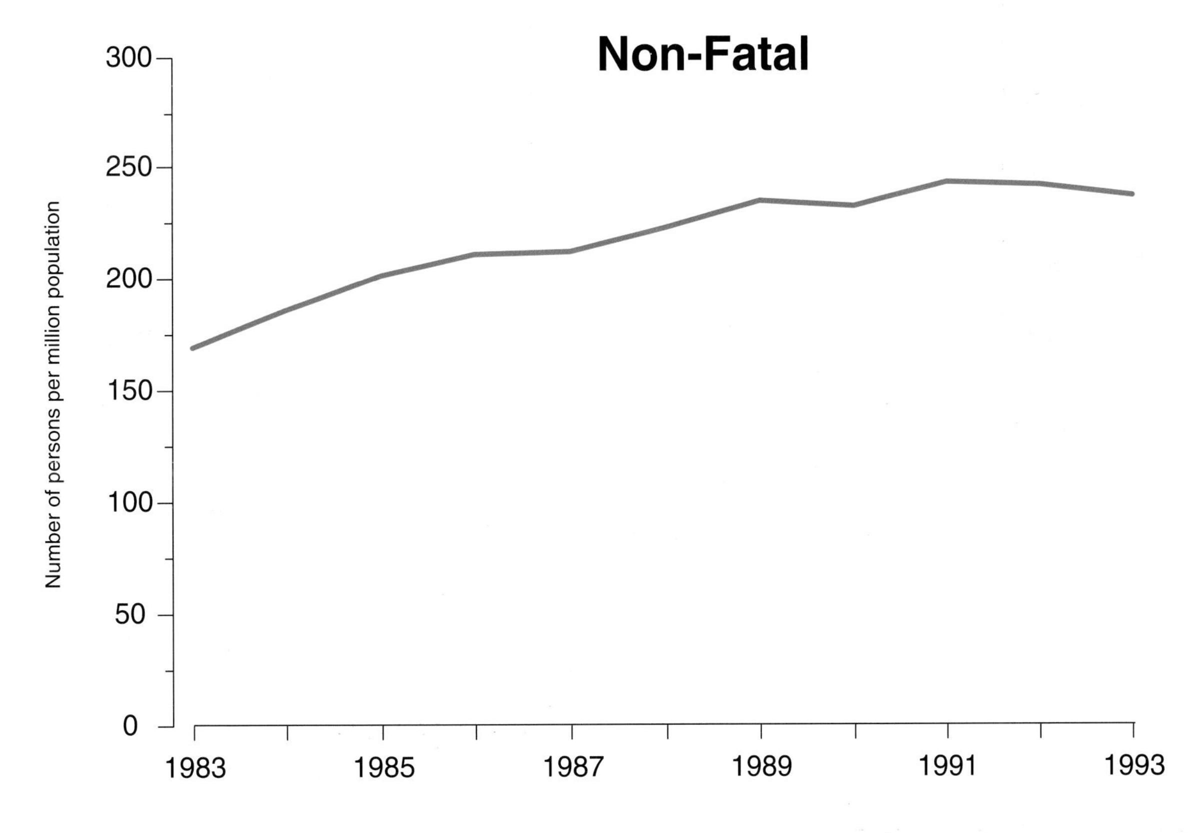

Source: Home Office Statistical Bulletin Issue 29/94

Figure AC5: Casualties from Fires†
by Age United Kingdom 1992

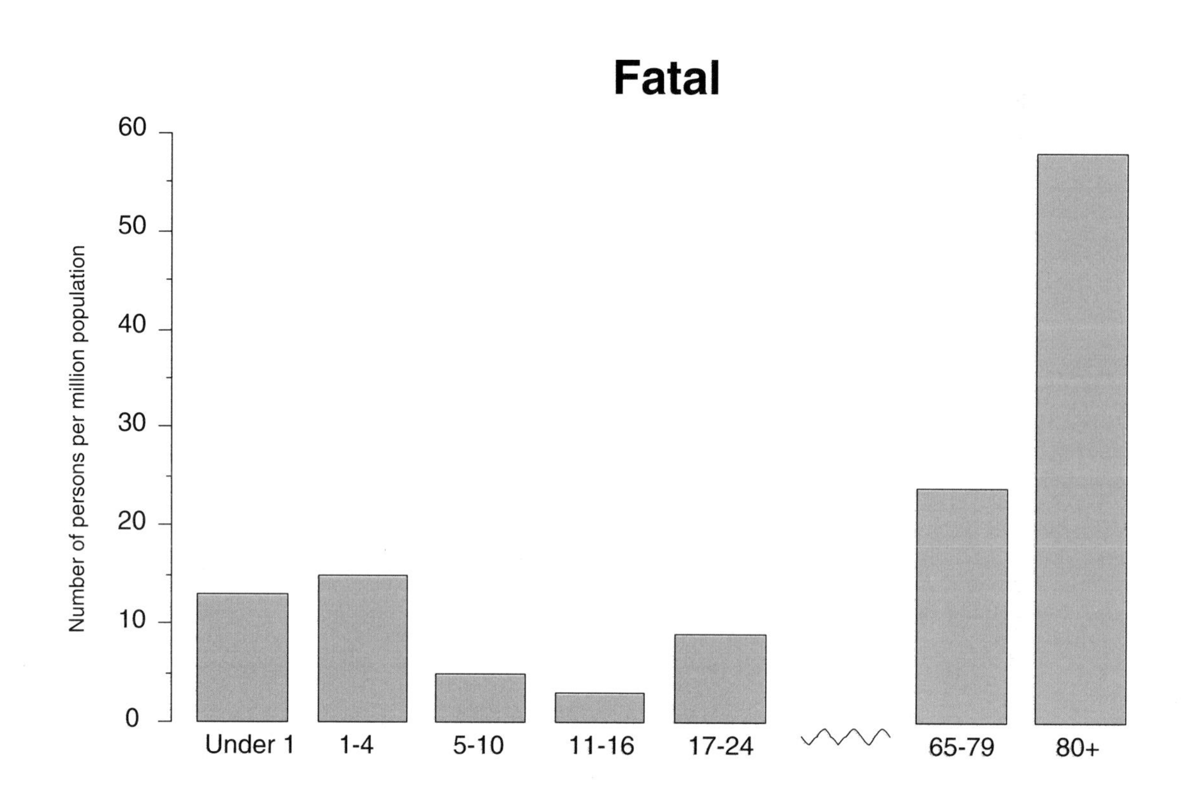

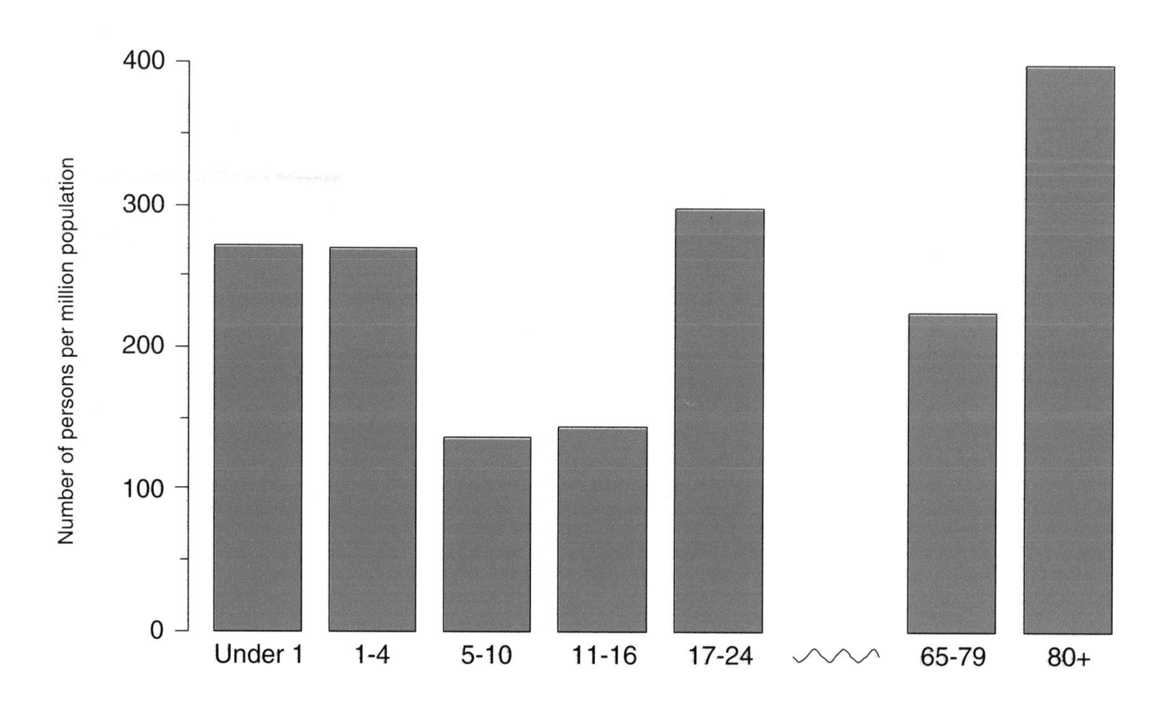

† Excludes fire brigade casualties
Source: Home Office Fire Statistics UK

Figure AC6: Households with a Smoke Alarm
by Age of Head of Household Great Britain 1991/92

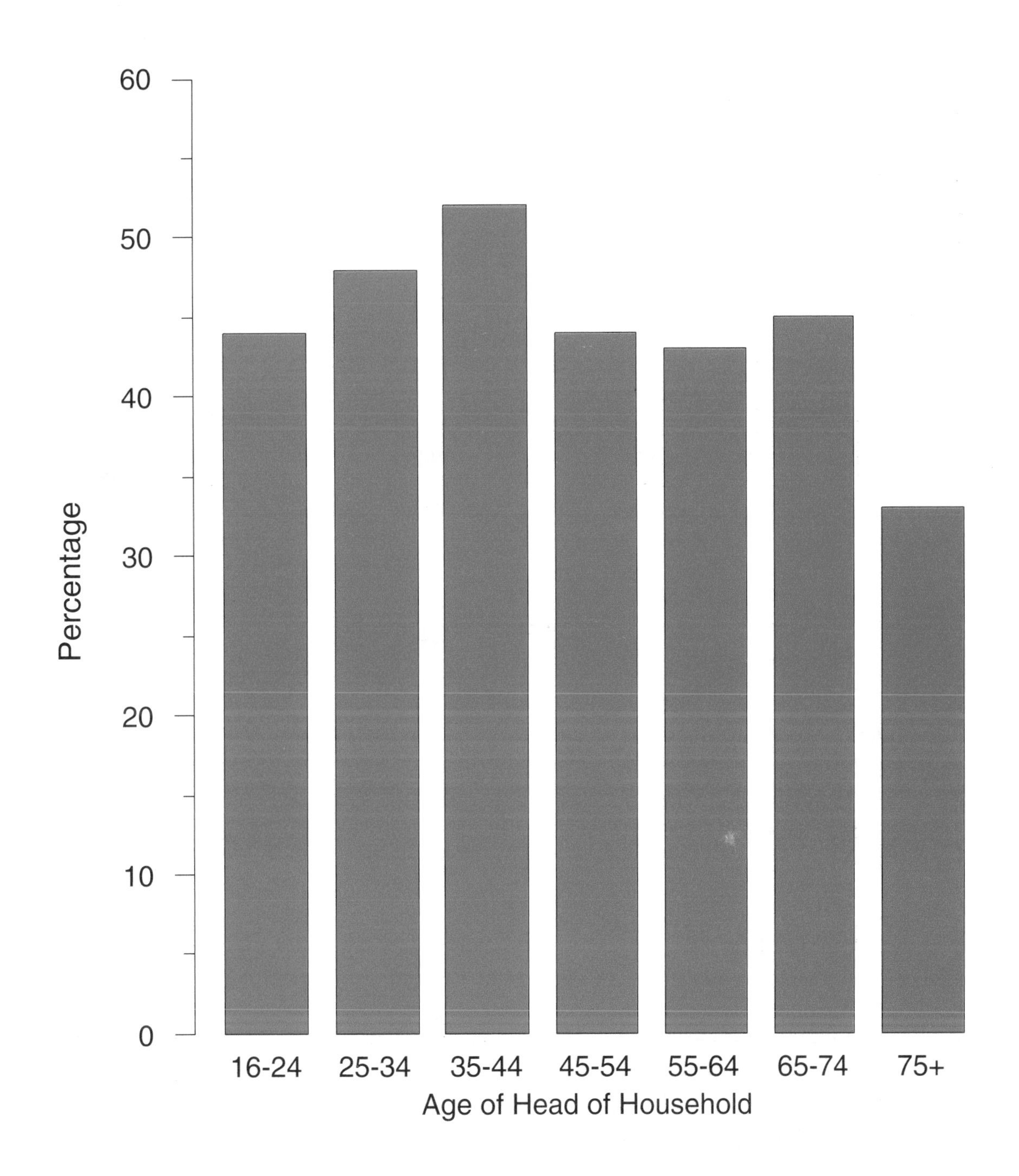

Source: OPCS Omnibus Survey

Figure AC7: Non Fatal Home Accidents
by Type & Age United Kingdom 1992

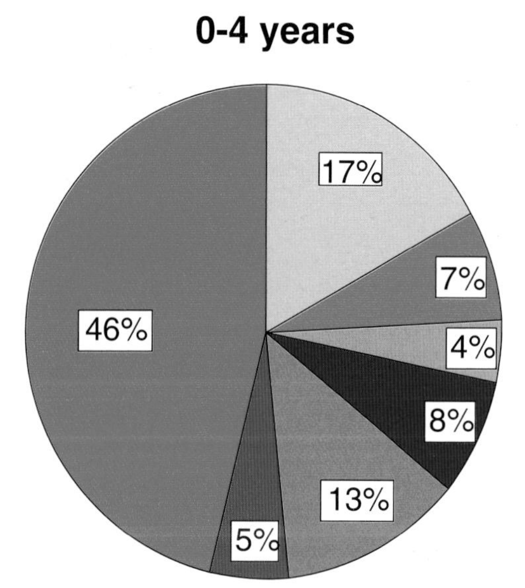

Estimated total accidents 623,000

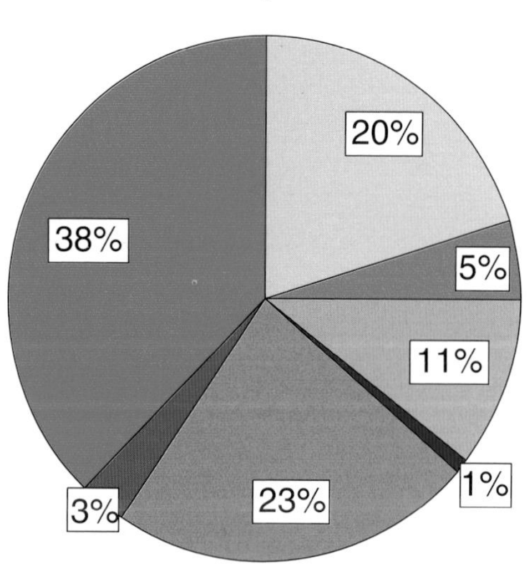

Estimated total accidents 400,000

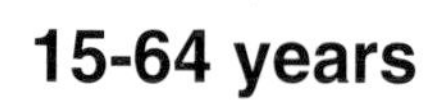

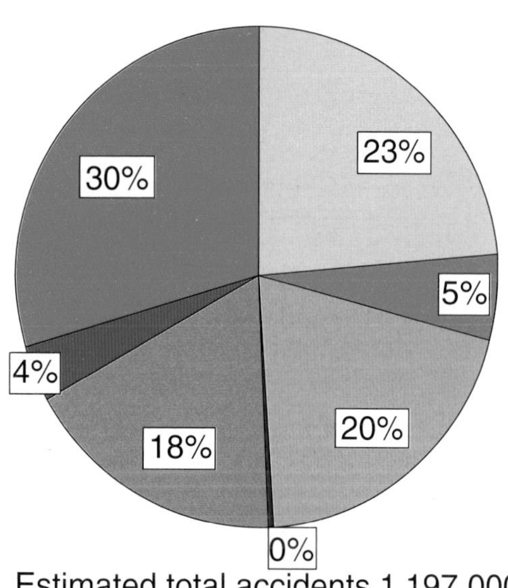

Estimated total accidents 1,197,000

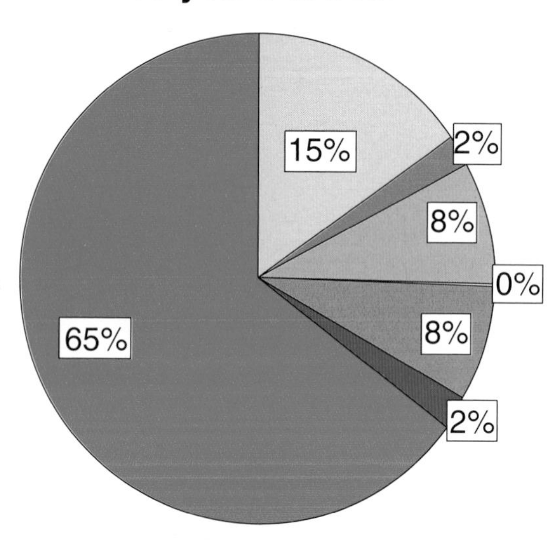

Estimated total accidents 318,000

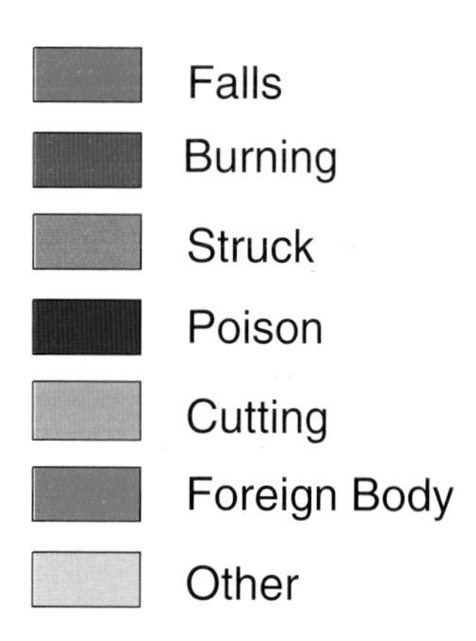

Source: DTI Home & Leisure Accident Research 1992 Data

Table AC1 *Mortality from external causes by selected place of birth, age 20–69 England and Wales, 1979–83*

	Accidental poisoning				Fire			
	Men		Women		Men		Women	
	SMR	no.	SMR	no.	SMR	no.	SMR	no.
Indian subcontinent	128	*42*	79	*12*	121	*15*	214	*15*
Caribbean Commonwealth	157	*24*	160	*15*	248	*16*	191	*8*
African Commonwealth	130	*19*	132	*7*	98	*4*	313	*7*

SMR – Standardised mortality ratios for England and Wales=100
no. – number of deaths

Source: Raleigh and Balajaran (1990)

Table AC2 *Road accidents and casualties 1981–1993 GB*

ACCIDENTS

	1981/85 average	1991	1992	1993
Accident rate[1]	84	57	56	55
Fatal & serious accidents as proportion of all accidents	27%	20%	19%	18%

CASUALTIES

	1981/85 average	1991	1992	1993	% change from 81/85 to 93
Under 16					
Fatal casualties	563	383	310	306	–45.6
Casualty rate[2]	*431*	*398*	*390*	*372*	*–13.6*
16–59					
Fatal casualties	3,549	2,914	2,752	2,382	–32.9
Casualty rate	*734*	*694*	*692*	*676*	*–7.9*
60 and over					
Fatal casualties	1,470	1,249	1,156	1,111	–24.4
Casualty rate	*296*	*287*	*277*	*281*	*–5.0*

1 Accident rate per 100 million vehicle kilometres
2 Casualty rate per 100 thousand population

Source: DoT Road Accidents GB 1992 The Casualty Report
DoT Road Accidents GB 1993 The Casualty Report

Table AC3 *Distance travelled per person per year by mode and by age and sex 1991/93 (miles)*

	Children	**Men**			**Women**		
	Under 16	**16–29**	**30–59**	**60+**	**16–29**	**30–59**	**60+**
Walk	225	245	191	215	247	212	167
Bicycle	35	110	63	36	21	18	5
Car user	3,089	6,764	9,196	3,885	5,055	5,463	2,276
Motorcycle	1	131	104	10	21	16	2

Source: DoT National Travel Survey

Table AC4 *Death rates from accidents in the home by age and sex, E&W 1992 (per million population)*

	0–5	**5–14**	**15–44**	**45–64**	**65–74**	**75+**	**All ages**
Male	47	11	42	65	132	515	69
Female	30	6	16	33	94	611	74

Figure in italics based on less than 20 deaths

Source: OPCS Series DH4 no 18 Table 5

DATA SOURCES

The sources were selected on the basis of the following criteria

used for setting HON target
used by Department for monitoring
national general population data
published data
contains socio-demographic information
trend data available

It can be seen from the matrix that behaviours such as smoking and alcohol are well researched nationally whereas other areas are not. This does not mean that research has not been conducted but that national data sources are not available.

It should be noted that where source references are given in italics the data have been collected but are not published.

Further Research

Behaviours that would seem to require more research include screening for cancer, suicide and drug misuse. This last area will be covered to some extent by the publication of results from the OPCS Surveys of Psychiatric Morbidity in Great Britain. A series of reports are due to be published throughout 1995/6.

In terms of socio-demographic data, ethnic group and people with disabilities are two areas where research is available but these are generally small scale localised studies and there is no comprehensive large scale data source. The publication of further results of the HEA Survey of Black and Minority Ethnic Communities and the Policy Studies Institute's 4th National Survey of Ethnic Minorities will add to the data base on ethnic groups.

Another important source of data will be the Health Education Monitoring Survey which is being conducted for the Health Education Authority by OPCS. This survey covers the main elements of health related behaviour. First results are due in 1996. The Health and Lifestyle Survey (UK) carried out in 1993 is expected to be published in 1996.

MATRIX OF SOURCES

Figures refer to Reference numbers

Behaviours	Age	Sex	Trend	Region	Scotland	Wales	Northern Ireland	Social Class	Employment Status	Marital Status	Household Type	Ethnic Origin	Disability	Other Sources
% of food energy from:														
total fat	30 (GB)	30 (GB)	25 (GB)	26	26	26	*	30 (GB)	30 (GB)	_30_	26 (GB)	*	*	40, 26A
saturated fatty acids	"	"	"	"	"	"		"	"	"	"	*	*	"
consumption of specific foods:														
milk, spreads, fruit/veg, bread	35	35	25 (GB)	35	26	26	*	35	_35_	_35_	_35_	*	*	30, 40
% of men drinking > 21 units and														
of women drinking > 14 units/week	34 (GB)/47	34 (GB)/47	34 (GB)	34	34	34	*	34 (GBSEG)	34 (GB)	34 (GB)	_34_	*	*	35, 22, 17, 31, 56
casualties/fatalities in road														
accidents involving alcohol	9 (GB)	*	9 (GB)	9	9	_9_	*	*	*	*	*	*	*	
% engaging in vigorous activity														
at least 3x20 mins/week	35	35	35/36	35	*	_18_	28	56	_35_	_35_	_35_	_12_	*	61
% engaging in moderate activity:														
% less 1x30 mins/week	23	23	*	_61_	*	*	*	13	13	*	*	_12_	*	
% at least 5x30 mins/week	"	"	*	"	*	"	"	"	"	"	"	"	*	
prevalence of cigarette smoking														
among men and women 16+	6	6	6	34	34	34	*	34 (GB)	34 (GB)	34 (GB)	_34_	12	*	58, 35, 22 18, 15
prevalence of cigarette smoking														
among boys & girls 11–15	48	48	48	48	47	47	*	17	NA	NA	*	17	*	
% of pregnant women smokers														
who give up while pregnant	36 (GB)	NA	36 (GB)	_36_	_36_	36	*	36 (GB)	_36_	_36_	*	*	*	16, 52, 50
% of women aged 50–64 taking up														
invitation to breast screening	*	NA	*	2	*	*	*	*	*	*	*	*	*	_17A_, 57
% of women taking up invitation														
to cervical screening	3	NA	*	3	*	*	*	*	*	*	*	3	*	_17A_, 22
prevalence of sunburn	43	43	*	43	43	43	*	43	43	43	43	*	*	
overall suicide rate	37 (EW)	37 (EW)	44 (EW)	39	*	39	*	45	*	45	*	54/55	*	53
suicide rate among severely mentally ill	*	*	*	*	*	*	*	*	*	*	*	*	*	49
use of condoms in past year	59 (GB)	59 (GB)	33 (GB)	_59_	_59_	59	*	59 (GB)	*	59 (GB)	*	*	*	42, _12_, 17A
age at first intercourse	59 (GB)	59 (GB)	*	*	*	*	*	59 (GB)	*	_59_	*	59 (GB)	*	
no. of sexual partners	59 (GB)	59 (GB)	*	*	*	*	*	59 (GB)	*	59 (GB)	*	_59_	*	11, 27, 24 46, 14
no. of conceptions under age 16	29 (EW)	NA	29 (EW)	29 (EW)	*	29	*	*	*	*	*	*	*	
% of injecting drug misusers														
sharing injecting equipment	52	52	7/52	*	*	*	*	*	*	*	*	*	*	9, _44_, 45
accidental deaths	37 (EW)	37 (EW)	37 (EW)	39	*	39	*	*	*	*	*	*	*	
casualties/deaths in:														
road accidents	37/9 (GB)	37 (EW)	9 (GB)	39	*	9	*	*	*	*	*	1	*}	
fires	37/20 (GB)	37/20 (UK)	21 (EW)	*	21	*	*	*	*	*	*	*	*}	
% households with smoke alarm	41	_41_	41	41	41	41	*	41	*	*	41	*	*}	51, 19, 53
casualties/deaths in home accidents	38/10/32	38 (EW) 32	10	*	*	*	*	*	*	*	*	*	*}	

REFERENCES

Department of Health. Health of the Nation A strategy for health in England, London HMSO 1992 (CM1986)

Department of Health. Specification of National Indicators. DH 1992

Numbers refer to the matrix of sources

1 Balarajan R and Bulusu L. Mortality among immigrants in England and Wales, 1979–83 in Mortality and Geography OPCS Series DS no. 9, London 1990

2 DH. Breast Cancer Screening 1992–93 Summary Information from Form KC62 England

3 DH. Cervical Cytology 1992–93. Summary Information from Form KC53 England

4 DH. Ethnicity and Health, DH 1993

5 DH. Report on Health and Social Subjects 46, Nutritional Aspects of Cardiovascular Diseases Report of the Cardiovascular Review Group. Committee on Medical Aspects of Food Policy. London HMSO 1994

6 DH. Statistical Bulletin 1994/14. Statistics on smoking England 1974 to 1993

7 Donoghoe M, Stimson G, Dolan K. Syringe Exchange in England An Overview, The Tufnell Press 1992

8 DoT. National Travel Survey 91/93 London HMSO 1994

9 DoT. Road Accidents Great Britain 1993 The Casualty Report London HMSO 1994.

10 DTI. Home and Leisure Accident Research 1992 Data, DTI 1994

11 HEA. AIDS Research in Gay Bars Report on a Series of Quantitative Surveys, HEA 1993

12 HEA. Black and Minority Ethnic Groups in England, HEA 1994

13 HEA. Health Update – Physical Activity, HEA London 1995

14 HEA. Health Update – Sexual Health, HEA 1994

15 HEA. Health Update No.2 Smoking, HEA 1991

16 HEA. Smoking and Pregnancy Research 1992–1993

17 HEA. Tomorrow's Young Adults, HEA 1992

17A HEA. Health and Lifestyle Survey, HEA 1992

18 Health Promotion Wales. Health related behaviours in Wales, 1985–1993 findings from the Health in Wales Surveys. Technical report no. 8. Health Promotion Wales 1994

19 Higginson I. Health of the Nation Accident Targets; What Further Research is Needed ? London DH 1995

20 Home Office Fire Statistics UK 1992

21 Home Office Statistical Bulletin – Summary Fire Statistics UK 1993 Issue 29/94

22 HPRT. The Health and Lifestyle Survey – Seven Years On, Dartmouth Publishing Company 1993

23 Killoran A, Fentem P, Casperson C, (eds). Moving On. International perspectives on promoting physical activity, HEA London 1995.

24 LRC. The Durex Reports 1991 and 1994, Durex Publications LRC Products Ltd

25 MAFF. National Food Survey 1990, London HMSO 1991. GB.

26 MAFF. National Food Survey 1993, London HMSO 1994. GB.

26A Mills A & Tyler H. Food and Nutrient Intakes of British Infants Aged 6–12 Months, London HMSO 1992

27 MRC/DH. Project Sigma The Sexual Lifestyles of Gay and Bisexual Men in England and Wales, London HMSO 1992

28 Northern Ireland Health and Activity Survey, Belfast HMSO 1994

29 OPCS. Conception Series FM1 no 21

30 OPCS. The Dietary and Nutritional Survey of British Adults (1986/7), London HMSO 1990

31 OPCS. Drinking in E&W in the late 1980's, London HMSO

32 OPCS. General Household Survey 1989 London HMSO 1991 (Series GHS no 20)

33 OPCS. General Household Survey 1991 London HMSO 1993 (Series GHS no 22)

34 OPCS. General Household Survey 1992 London HMSO 1994 (Series GHS no 23)

35 OPCS. Health Survey for England 1993, London HMSO 1995.

36 OPCS. Infant Feeding 1990 London HMSO 1992

37 OPCS. Mortality Statistics Series DH2 no 19

38 OPCS. Mortality Statistics Series DH4 no 18

39 OPCS. Mortality Statistics Series DH5 no 18

40 OPCS. The National Diet and Nutrition Survey children aged 1 to 4 years, London HMSO 1995

41 OPCS. National Fire Safety Week and Domestic Fire Safety, London HMSO 1994

42 OPCS. Omnibus Survey 1990–1994

43 OPCS. Omnibus Survey October 1993. J Melia and A Bulman. Sunburn and tanning in a British population, Journal of Public Health Medicine 1995 vol 17 pp225–229.

44 OPCS. Population Trends no 69 Trends in suicide deaths in England and Wales London HMSO 1992

45 OPCS. Population Trends no 71 Suicide deaths in England and Wales trends in factors associated with suicide deaths London HMSO 1993

46 OPCS. Population Trends no 74 Teenage conceptions and fertility in England and Wales 1971–1991. London HMSO 1993

47 OPCS. Smoking among Secondary School Children in 1992. London HMSO 1993

48 OPCS. Smoking among Secondary School Children in England 1993. London HMSO 1994

49 OPCS. Surveys of Psychiatric Morbidity in Great Britain Bulletin No. 1, OPCS 1994, and Report 1, HMSO 1995

50 OPCS. Why children start smoking. London HMSO 1990

51 Public Health Information Strategy – Improving information on accidents, DH 1993

52 PHLS, DH, Institute of Child Health. Unlinked Anonymous HIV Prevalence Monitoring Programme England and Wales, DH 1995

53 Smaje C. Health, Race and Ethnicity. Kings Fund Institute 1995

55 Soni Raleigh V, Balarajan R. Suicide and self burning among Indians and West Indians in England and Wales. British Journal of Psychiatry 1992; 161 365–8

55 Soni Raleigh V, Bulusu L, Balarajan R. Suicides among immigrants from the Indian sub-continent. British Journal of Psychiatry 1990; 156 46–50

56 The Sports Council and Health Education Authority. Allied Dunbar National Fitness Survey – main findings, Sports Council. London 1992

57 Trent RHA NHS breast screening programme review 1993

58 Wald N. & Nicholaides-Bouman A. eds. UK Smoking Statistics (Tobacco Advisory Council) Oxford Oxford University Press, 1991

59 Wellings K, Field J, Johnson A, Wadsworth J. Sexual Behaviour in Britain Penguin Books 1994.

Not yet published

60 HEA Health and Lifestyle Survey 1993, HEA

61 HEA Physical Activity Matters across the Regions, HEA

62 Health Survey for England 1994, DH

63 National Diet and Nutrition Survey – adults aged 65+ Fieldwork 1995, DH and MAFF

Figures are percentages

RHA	North	Yorkshire	North West	Mersey	West Midlands	Trent	East Anglia	Oxford	North West Thames	North East Thames	South East Thames	South West Thames	Wessex	South West
DIET - MEN														
Usual fat spread: butter/hard marg.	21	18	19	25	21	16	22	22	27	30	23	24	24	25
Usual milk: whole milk	40	42	44	41	39	40	42	35	40	44	42	35	44	42
Fruit at least once a day	35	39	38	42	39	44	49	43	47	45	44	47	41	50
Veg/salad at least once a day	55	64	57	63	55	61	70	68	64	68	68	71	68	69
Bread more than once a day	50	40	49	39	42	42	36	31	34	34	28	34	40	33
DIET - WOMEN														
Usual fat spread: butter/hard marg.	27	21	23	21	20	17	21	19	25	27	21	23	22	22
Usual milk: whole milk	35	34	39	35	35	32	32	30	32	39	34	30	36	36
Fruit at least once a day	48	48	47	50	50	53	61	54	63	55	56	59	56	59
Veg/salad at least once a day	56	65	62	64	70	64	72	74	74	68	71	75	71	73
Bread more than once a day	39	30	37	31	33	30	29	26	29	27	23	30	30	26

Sample sizes for RHAs in Health Survey 1993
Bases for each category above may be very slightly smaller because of non-response. See report of Health Survey 1993

Men	*536*	*610*	*653*	*397*	*814*	*729*	*357*	*412*	*551*	*534*	*563*	*500*	*505*	*528*
Women	*642*	*707*	*786*	*485*	*902*	*819*	*402*	*477*	*598*	*607*	*692*	*566*	*575*	*622*

REGIONAL TABLES STANDARDISED MORTALITY RATIOS (1992/93)

RHA	North	Yorkshire	North West	Mersey	West Midlands	Trent	East Anglia	Oxford	North West Thames	North East Thames	South East Thames	South West Thames	Wessex	South West
SUICIDE - MEN														
Suicide (SMR)	88	97	105	115	96	92	94	89	106	100	107	89	82	122
Undetermined injury	123	107	74	78	124	118	127	90	93	78	91	82	95	113
SUICIDE - WOMEN														
Suicide (SMR)	70	93	87	88	97	103	119	102	106	95	114	91	90	124
Undetermined injury	104	118	97	105	126	110	120	82	92	*47*	67	85	102	133
ACCIDENTS - MEN														
All accidents (E800 - E949)	106	98	103	108	92	101	88	83	83	93	93	99	109	112
Motor vehicle accidents (E810 - E819)	114	104	121	119	79	88	86	81	103	91	111	95	86	90
Falls (E880 - E888)	127	94	95	101	90	115	77	75	56	98	90	116	91	137
ACCIDENTS - WOMEN														
All accidents (E800 - E949)	119	99	100	108	95	91	81	76	91	110	94	112	75	113
Motor vehicle accidents (E810 - E819)	117	104	120	122	94	79	91	97	107	99	95	88	87	97
Falls (E880 - E888)	136	100	101	109	81	82	56	55	89	119	103	133	66	128

Source: OPCS Series DH5 no 18 (SMRs in italics based on fewer than 20 deaths)

GLOSSARY

The glossary includes references to general data sources. Notes referring to specific surveys can be found at the end of the relevant section.

General Household Survey (GHS)

The General Household Survey (GHS) is a continuous survey which has been running since 1971 and is based each year on a sample of the general population aged 16 and over resident in private (that is, non-institutional) households in Great Britain. The fieldwork year runs from April to March. During the period April 1992 to March 1993 (the 1992 survey) 19,079 people were interviewed. The data from this survey are not age adjusted.

Health Survey For England

The Health Survey is commissioned by the Department of Health and is designed to provide better and more regular information on various aspects of people's health. Its initial focus has been on cardiovascular disease and related conditions. 1993 was the third year of the Health Survey and the first in which fieldwork was carried out throughout the whole year. A total of 16,569 adults aged 16+ resident in private (that is, non-institutional) households were interviewed between January and December of 1993.

The Office of Population Censuses and Surveys (OPCS)

The Office of Population Censuses and Surveys (OPCS) is the office of the Registrar General for England and Wales. Its responsibilities include

- the registration of births, deaths and marriages
- the preparation of population and medical statistics
- the census of population

In addition, OPCS has a Social Survey Division which covers Scotland as well as England and Wales. Social Survey Division carries out sample surveys of individuals and households to provide information on subjects such as health, housing, employment and many other matters of public concern.

Omnibus Survey

An omnibus survey is a continuous survey which collects data on a modular basis. The modules do not have to be related to each other and can be included for different clients. Modules can have a single entry in the survey or can be repeated at regular intervals. Omnibus surveys are useful for providing quick answers to questions of immediate interest and information on topics too brief to require a full survey.

The OPCS Omnibus Survey is a monthly survey for government departments and public bodies. It conducts interviews with around 2000 adults aged 16+ each month based on a representative random sample of Great Britain. Results are presented in the form of a floppy disc and are available from OPCS with the agreement of the sponsor.

Proportional Mortality Ratios (PMRs)

The PMR is calculated as follows

PMR=Observed deaths/Expected deaths x 100

The expected deaths from a particular cause are computed by applying the proportion of total deaths from that cause in the comparison or general population to the total deaths in the group of interest. Care should be taken when interpreting PMRs since the relative frequency of other causes of death can affect the proportional mortality for the cause of interest. As a result, an observed excess for one cause of death in the exposed group may represent a true increased risk, but may also simply represent a deficit of deaths from other causes.

Secular Trends – trends over time

Social Class

Social class within the context of statistical analysis usually refers to the grouping of people according to their occupation based on the Registrar General's Classification of Occupations (1980).

All occupations are classified into five main groups, the five 'social classes'. Social class III and IV are further sub-divided into non-manual and manual groups. In presentation, class IV is often left as one group.

I Professional occupations
II Intermediate occupations (now called managerial and technical)
IIIN Non-manual skilled occupations
IIIM Manual skilled occupations
IV Partly skilled occupations
V Unskilled occupations

Within this classification, members of the armed forces are classified as a separate group.

Social class can be based on the individual's occupation or that of the head of household. The latter option is more common among the main surveys used for this overview. This difference is particularly important when looking at the social class of women who are less likely to be the head of household.

In addition to the 'social class' classification 'socio-economic group' is also used in particular in the General Household Survey. This further grouping takes into account position as well as skill level.

Standardised Mortality Ratio

Age standardisation is a method of adjusting a set of data to compensate for the effects of different age distributions within the populations being compared. It is possible to standardise by any variable which is thought to have an effect on the overall estimates.

The Standardised Mortality Ratio (SMR) is the measure most widely used in this country to compare mortality rates in different population groupings because it takes account of any differences in the age and sex structures. The SMR is derived as follows

$$\frac{\text{Observed Number of Deaths}}{\text{Expected Number of Deaths}} \times 100$$

The observed number is the actual number of deaths in the geographical area or sub-group of the population. The expected number of deaths is calculated by applying the age and sex specific mortality rates for the population as a whole to the population of the area or sub-group.

For example, in the case of English data the SMR for England is 100. If the population of a Health Authority demonstrates a mortality rate which is greater than the English average (after taking account of any differences in the age and sex structure), then the Health Authority's SMR will be greater than 100.

Printed in the UK for The Stationery Office
Dd 303841, C8, 04/97